SOUPS COOKBOOK

Over 50+ Delicious Homemade Soup Recipes

(A Collection of Easy, Simple and Delicious Asian Soups)

Charlene Arceneaux

Published by Alex Howard

© **Charlene Arceneaux**

All Rights Reserved

Soups Cookbook: Over 50+ Delicious Homemade Soup Recipes (A Collection of Easy, Simple and Delicious Asian Soups)

ISBN 978-1-990169-36-6

All rights reserved. No part of this guide may be reproduced in any form without permission in writing from the publisher except in the case of brief quotations embodied in critical articles or reviews.

Legal & Disclaimer

The information contained in this book is not designed to replace or take the place of any form of medicine or professional medical advice. The information in this book has been provided for educational and entertainment purposes only.

The information contained in this book has been compiled from sources deemed reliable, and it is accurate to the best of the Author's knowledge; however, the Author cannot guarantee its accuracy and validity and cannot be held liable for any errors or omissions. Changes are periodically made to this book. You must consult your doctor or get professional medical advice before using any of the suggested remedies, techniques, or information in this book.

Table of contents

PART 1 1

INTRODUCTION 2

CHICKEN GNOCCHI SOUP 4
CHICKEN AND BEAN SOUP 5
EASY CHICKEN NOODLE SOUP 6
CHICKEN VEGETABLE SOUP 7
CHICKEN AND POTATO SOUP 8
CHICKEN AND CARROT SOUP 9
TORTILLA CHICKEN SOUP 10
CHICKEN RICE SOUP 11
CARROT CHICKEN NOODLE SOUP 12
CHILI CHICKEN SOUP 13
CHICKEN BACON SOUP 14
CHICKEN AND PASTA SOUP 15
CHICKEN BARLEY SOUP 16
MUSHROOM CHICKEN SOUP 17
CHICKEN LENTIL SOUP 18
ADOBO CHICKEN SOUP 19
THAI CHICKEN SOUP 20
PARMESAN CHICKEN SOUP 21
SLOW COOKER CHICKEN BROTH 22
CHICKEN STOCK 23
YOU CAN HAVE SOUP ANYTIME 24
CUCUMBER SOUP 26
BROCCOLI SOUP 27
BUTTERNUT SQUASH SAGE SOUP 28
POTATO LEEK SOUP 29
TOMATO SOUP 30
ROSEMARY WHITE BEAN SOUP 31
CARROT AND BEET SOUP 32
CARROT AND POTATO 33

Tomato And Basil Soup	34
Spiced Pumpkin Soup	35
Cherry Tomato Soup	36
Tasty Vegetable Soup	37
Quick Watermelon Gazpacho	38
Cauliflower Soup	39
Pea Soup	40
Roasted Carrot Soup	41
Cauliflower Pear Soup	42
Celery Soup	43
Abc Soup	44
Abalone And Peas Soup	45
Abalone And Chicken Soup	46
Asparagus Soup	47
Bean Sprouts And Egg Drop Soup	48
Bird's Nest Soup	49
Cabbage And Prawn Soup	50
Cabbage Soup	51
Celery Soup	52
Chicken And Sweet Corn Soup	53
Chicken And Ham Soup	54
Chicken And Mushroom Soup	55
Chicken Chowder	56
Chicken Soup With Egg	57
Chicken Soup With Fried Noodles	58
Crab Meat Soup	59
Cucumber And Minced Chicken Soup	60
Duck And Orange Peel Soup	61
Duck And Salted Vegetable Soup	62
Egg Soup	63
Fish Chowder	64
Fish Soup	65
Lettuce And Egg Drop Soup	66
Lettuce And Shrimp Soup	67
Mixed Vegetables Soup	68
Mushroom And Peas Soup	69

Mushroom Soup	70
Prawn Soup Rice	71
Peas And Egg Drop Soup	72
Pigeon Soup	73
Roast Pork And Mushroom Soup	74
Shark's Fin Soup	75
Spinach Soup	76
Sweet Corn With Pork And Egg Shreds Soup	77
Tomato And Egg Soup	78
Wan Ton Soup	79
Watercress Soup	80
Whole Chicken With Bird's Nest Soup	81
Creamy Spinach Soup	82
Tip	83
Pumpkin Soup	84
Tip	85
Cream Of Wild Mushroom Soup	86
Tip	87
Spinach Soup	88
Tip	89
Shirred Squash Soup	90
Frothy Cannellini Soup	92
Tip	93
Simple Coconut & Bean Soup	94
Lightly Spiced Carrot Soup	96
Tip	97
Quick Gazpacho	98
Rich Tomato Soup With Pesto	99
Tip	100
Spicy Pasta Soup	101
Tip	102
Hearty Mushroom Soup	103
PART 2	**105**
Quick Chilled Pea Soup	106
Black Bean Soup	108

- Caramelized Onion And Shiitake Soup With Gruyère–Blue Cheese Toasts 110
- Soup: 110
- Lemon, Orzo, And Meatball Soup 113
- Posole (Tomatillo, Chicken, And Hominy Soup) 115
- Hot And Sour Shrimp Soup 117
- Black Bean Soup With Chorizo And Lime 119
- Cauliflower Soup With Shiitakes 121
- Broccoli-Cheddar Soup 123
- Two-Mushroom Velouté 125
- Pozole 127
- Garnishes: 128
- Red Lentil-Pumpkin Soup 130
- Thai Chicken Soup 132
- Beef Dumpling Soup 134
- Spicy Coconut Shrimp Soup 136
- Roasted SQuash Soup With Sage 138
- Baby Carrot Soup 140
- Toppings: 140
- Cheeseburger Soup 142
- Optional: 142
- Butternut SQuash-Parsnip Soup 144
- Optional: 145
- Zucchini Soup 146
- Garnishes: 146
- Roasted Red Pepper Soup With Pesto Croutons 148
- Avocado Soup With Citrus-Shrimp Relish 150
- Soup: 150
- Red Pepper-Cauliflower Soup 152
- Spicy Tomato And White Bean Soup 154
- Green Onion Egg Drop Soup 156
- Roasted Red Pepper Soup 158
- Southwestern Chicken Soup 160
- Thai Coconut Soup 162
- Tortilla Soup With Chorizo And Turkey Meatballs 164
- Curried Cauliflower Soup 166
- Classic Chicken Noodle Soup 169

Turkey Meatball Soup With Greens	171
Mini Meatball Minestrone	173
Coconut Laksa With Shrimp	176
Chicken-And-Prosciutto Tortelloni Soup	179
Southern Italian Chicken Soup	181
Amish Style Chicken And Corn Soup	183
Chicken And Dumplings Soup	185
Soup:	185
Dumplings:	185
Soup:	186
Dumplings:	186
Debra's Cauliflower Soup	187

Part 1

Introduction

The entire world is officially in love with soup. There is no country or town or village under the sun where you'll go and not find at least a kitchen with a pot of soup cooking. What is with us and soup? We all have one thing in common-the desire to feel loved and to be loved. And a bowl of warm soup provides just that. It warms our heart, comforts our spirits, and quiets our souls.

When I say soup I don't mean any soup. Powdered or canned or bottle soups are convenient and save time, but they'll never give you that satisfaction, comfort, and nutrition you get from home cooked soup.

There is something special about a pot of soup simmering in the kitchen. The warmth it creates in the house. The way it perfumes the air with sweet scent. The way it makes you feel everything is going to be fine. You can never get this from store bought soup. It's why I love to cook my own soup. And I can always have control over what I can or not include in my soup.

When you prepare soup from home, you not only get the comfort and satisfaction it gives, you also nourish your body with vital nutrients found in the veggies, fruits, meats, and other ingredients used.

Our love affair with soup is growing stronger and deeper by the day. With the advent of slow cookers, anyone even the busiest person or laziest cook can soothe their souls with a comforting bowl of chicken soup.

Slow cookers are convenient and cheap to use. They take less energy, turn cheap cuts of meat tender, and you may leave the food cooking while you go for work or take care of other responsibilities like playing with kids, taking your dog for a walk, taking care of your flowers.

If you can chop or slice or grate and can press buttons, you can make tasty soup in your slow cooker.

If you love chicken soup and was looking for a variety of recipes you can cook each day of the week, you have found the right book. If you are busy and normally don't get time to cook, but would always love to have something made from home in your slow cooker, these simple soups will meet you at your point of need. If you are a fan of soup and just looking for something to quench your thirst for soup, this book has variety of chicken soups to get you going.

Chicken Gnocchi Soup

Servings: 8

Prep: 10 minutes

Cook: 6 hours

Ingredients

- 1 pound chicken breast, boneless, skinless, and cut into bite size cubes
- 2 pounds pkg. potato gnocchi
- 2 cups vegetable mix (carrots, celery, onions)
- 5 ounces baby spinach, fresh
- 2 (12 ounces each) cans evaporated milk
- 3 garlic cloves, minced
- 4 cups chicken broth
- 6 slices bacon, diced
- 3 tablespoons cornstarch mixed with water
- 1 teaspoon poultry seasoning
- 1 teaspoon salt
- 1 teaspoon basil, dried

Preparation

- In the slow cooker, add chicken broth, vegetable mix, Italian seasoning, salt, poultry seasoning, and basil.
- Cover and cook for 5 hours on high.
- Stir in cornstarch paste, gnocchi, and evaporated milk.
- Cook covered for 1 hour on low.
- Add spinach and cook until wilted.
- Heat a skillet over medium-high. Add bacon and cook until crispy. Drain off excess fat and stir into the soup.
- Taste and season as desired.

Chicken And Bean Soup

Servings: 8

Prep: 15 minutes

Cook: 7 hours

Ingredients
- 3 chicken breasts, skinless, boneless, and cut into bite size cubes
- 410g tin black beans
- 450g tin chili beans
- 340g tins drained sweet corn kernels
- 30g packet taco seasoning
- 225g passata
- 1 onion, chopped
- 350ml beer

Preparation
- In the slow cooker, add all ingredients and cover. Cook on low for 7 hours.

Easy Chicken Noodle Soup

Servings: 6

Prep: 10 minutes

Cook: 8 hours and 30 minutes

Ingredients
- 350g egg noodles, cooked
- 4 chicken breasts, skinless, boneless, cut into bite size pieces
- 2 celery sticks, chopped
- 1 ½ Liters water
- 1 onion, chopped
- Salt, to taste
- Fresh ground black pepper, to taste

Preparation
- In the slow cooker, add all ingredients except noodles.
- Cover and cook for 8 hours on low.
- Add noodles, heat through and serve.

Chicken Vegetable Soup

Servings: 4

Prep: 10 minutes

Cook: 4 hours

Ingredients
- 1 pound chicken breast, skinless, boneless, cut into bite size cubes
- 5 cups chicken broth
- 1 cup broccoli, chopped
- ½ teaspoon kosher salt
- 2 teaspoons Worcestershire sauce
- 1 zucchini, finely chopped
- 2 celery stalks, finely chopped
- 1 onion, finely chopped
- 1 carrot, finely diced
- 2 garlic cloves, minced
- 1 bay leaf
- Salt, to taste
- Freshly ground black pepper, to taste

Preparation
- In the slow cooker, add all ingredients and cover.
- Cook on low for 7 hours.
- Taste and season as desired.

Chicken And Potato Soup

Servings: 4

Prep: 10 minutes

Cook: 2 hours

Ingredients

- 1 pound sweet potatoes, peeled, cubed
- 2 pounds chicken thighs, boneless
- 6 cups chicken broth
- ¼ cup parsley, fresh, minced
- 1 leek, sliced
- 1 yellow onion, peeled, chopped
- 2 bay leaves
- 6 celery ribs, chopped
- 6 carrots, peeled, finely chopped
- 1 teaspoon thyme, fresh
- 2 teaspoons salt
- 2 teaspoons black pepper, ground
- 2 tablespoons extra-virgin olive oil

Preparation

- In the slow cooker, add oil, chicken, salt, pepper, bay leaves, thyme, and broth.
- Cover and cook for 1 hour on low.
- Add all remaining ingredients except parsley.
- Cover and cook for 1 hour on low.
- Shred chicken into bite size pieces.
- Serve garnished with parsley.

Chicken And Carrot Soup

Servings: 8

Prep: 10 minutes

Cook: 8 hours

Ingredients
- 4 pounds whole chicken, giblets and neck removed
- 4 large carrots, peeled, finely chopped
- 1 bay leaf
- 1 yellow onion, chopped
- 3 celery stalks, chopped
- 2 tablespoons Italians parsley leaves, chopped
- 1 tablespoon kosher salt
- 1 tablespoon olive oil
- ½ teaspoon thyme, dried
- ½ teaspoon black pepper, freshly ground
- 8 cups of water

Preparation
- Add all ingredients into the slow cooker and cover.
- Cook on low for 8 hours.
- Remove chicken into a platter and cut into bite sizes pieces. Return chicken into the slow cooker.
- Heat through and serve.

Tortilla Chicken Soup

Servings: 8

Prep: 15 minutes

Cook: 8 hours

Ingredients

- 450g chicken, cooked cut into shreds
- 7 corn tortillas, cut into strips
- 400ml chicken stock
- 475ml water
- 280g sweet corn, frozen
- 100g jalapeno pepper, chopped
- 400g tin crushed tomatoes
- 352g Jar enchilada sauce
- 1 teaspoon chili powder
- ¼ teaspoon black pepper
- 1 teaspoon salt
- 1 teaspoon cumin
- 1 tablespoon coriander, chopped
- 1 onion, chopped
- 2 garlic cloves, minced
- 1 bay leaf

Preparation

- In the slow cooker, add all ingredients except tortilla.
- Cover and cook for 6 hours on low.
- Meanwhile, preheat your oven to 200^0 C.
- Sprinkle tortilla with oil and place on a baking tray.
- Place in the preheated oven and bake until crispy, about 10 minutes.
- Serve soup and top with tortillas.

Chicken Rice Soup

Serves: 8

Prep: 15 minutes

Cook: 4 hours

Ingredients

- 9 cups chicken broth
- 3 chicken breasts, excess fat removed, halved
- 1 cup brown rice, cooked
- 1 onion, chopped
- 1 bay leaf
- 3 garlic cloves, minced
- 3 carrots, chopped
- 3 celery stalks, finely chopped
- ½ teaspoon each; sage and rosemary
- 1 teaspoon thyme
- 2 teaspoons parsley
- 3 teaspoons salt

Preparation

- In the slow cooker, add chicken, carrots, celery, bay leaf, garlic clove, onion, salt, parsley, thyme, sage, rosemary, and chicken broth.
- Cover and cook for 4 hours on low.
- Remove chicken into a platter. Separate meat from bones, cut meat into small pieces, and return into the slow cooker.
- Add rice and cook until heated through.

Carrot Chicken Noodle Soup

Servings: 6

Prep: 20 minutes

Cook: 8 hours

Ingredients

- 3 ½ pounds roasting chicken
- 3 cups carrots, thinly sliced
- 3 cups egg noodles, cooked
- 2 bay leaves
- ½ teaspoon thyme, dried
- 8 cups chicken broth
- 1 onion, chopped
- 2 celery stalks, chopped
- 1 garlic clove, minced
- Salt, to taste
- Fresh ground black pepper, to taste

Preparation

- Add carrots, onion, celery, bay leaves, thyme, garlic, chicken broth, and chicken.
- Cook covered for 8 hours on low.
- Taste and season with salt and pepper.
- Remove and discard bay leaf.
- Remove chicken into a plate, separate meat from bones, and cut meat into shreds.
- Return meat into the slow cooker and add noodles.
- Cook until heated through.

Chili Chicken Soup

Servings: 6

Prep: 10 minutes

Cook: 8 hours and 10 minutes

Ingredients
- 1 teaspoon chili flakes, crushed
- 450g chicken thighs, skinless, boneless
- 1 Liter chicken stock
- 120ml water
- 100g mixed vegetables
- 400g tin chopped tomatoes
- 45g long grain rice
- ½ teaspoon each; salt and fresh ground black pepper
- 1 teaspoon basil leaves, dried
- 2 teaspoons garlic, minced
- 2 stalks celery, finely chopped
- 2 carrots, finely chopped
- 1 onion, finely chopped

Preparation
- Add all ingredients into the slow cooker except rice and mixed vegetables.
- Cover and cook for 7 hours on low.
- Add rice and vegetables, cook for 1 hour on high.
- Shred chicken and return into the soup.
- Taste and season as desired.

Chicken Bacon Soup

Servings: 6

Prep: 20 minutes

Cook: 4 hours

Ingredients

- 1 ½ pounds chicken thighs, skinless
- 4 cups chicken stock
- 4 bacon slices, diced
- 1 cup carrot, diced
- 1 cup celery, diced
- 2 cups baby spinach, chopped
- 2 cups leek, sliced
- 12 ounces baby potatoes, diced
- 2 teaspoons garlic herb seasoning
- ½ teaspoon black pepper, fresh
- 5 thyme sprigs
- ¾ teaspoon kosher salt

Preparation

- Heat a skillet over medium-high heat. Add bacon and cook for about 5 minutes or until crispy.
- Transfer bacon into a platter.
- In the same skillet, add chicken thighs and sprinkle with garlic herb seasoning.
- Cook until browned, about 8 minutes.
- Transfer into the slow cooker. Set aside.
- In the same skillet, add celery, leek and carrot. Cook for 5 minutes and transfer into the slow cooker.
- Add all remaining ingredients and cover. Cook for 4 hours on low.
- Transfer chicken into a platter and cut into bite size pieces.
- Return it into the pot, add spinach, and cook for a few minutes.

Chicken And Pasta Soup

Servings: 6

Prep: 5 minutes

Cook: 5 hours and 30 minutes

Ingredients
- 4 chicken thighs, skinless, boneless
- ½ cup small pasta
- ¼ cups flat-leaf parsley, chopped
- 2 bay leaves
- 2 garlic cloves, smashed
- 4 stalks celery, chopped
- 4 carrots, chopped
- 1 onion, chopped

Preparation
- Add water, chicken, carrot, onion, celery, garlic, bay leaf, and salt and pepper into the slow cooker.
- Cover and cook for 4 hours on high.
- Transfer chicken into a platter.
- Add pasta into the slow cooker. Cover and cook for 15 minutes or until al dente.
- Cut chicken into small pieces and return into the pot.
- Mix well and serve garnished with parsley.

Chicken Barley Soup

Servings: 5

Prep: 35 minutes

Cook: 8 hours

Ingredients

- ½ cup pearl barley
- 2 pounds fryer chicken, boneless, cut into bite size pieces
- 1 bay leaf
- ½ teaspoon each; dried sage, poultry seasoning, and pepper
- 1 teaspoon salt
- 2 quarts water
- 1 ½ cups onion, chopped
- 1 chicken bouillon cube

Preparation

- In the slow cooker, add all ingredients and cover. Cook for 8 hours on low.

Mushroom Chicken Soup

Servings: 4

Prep: 15 minutes

Cook: 7 hours

Ingredients
- 950g chicken breast, skinless
- 3 chicken stock pots
- 100g long grain rice
- 1 inch ginger piece, peeled, grated
- 2 bay leaves
- 4 garlic cloves
- 1 bunch spring onions, thinly sliced
- 1 teaspoon turmeric
- 2 Liters water

Preparation

- In the slow cooker, add chicken, mushrooms, ginger, garlic cloves, bay leaves, turmeric, chicken stock pot, and water. Stir to mix well. Cover and cook for 7 hours.
- Remove chicken into a platter. Separate meat from bones. Shred meat and return into the slow cooker.
- Add rice and cook until tender.
- Serve garnished with spring onions.

Chicken Lentil Soup

Servings: 6

Prep: 15 minutes

Cook: 4 hours

Ingredients
- 1 pound chicken, skinless, boneless
- 1 pound lentils, dried
- 7 ½ cups chicken broth
- 1 teaspoon each; onion powder, garlic powder
- 1 ½ teaspoons each; smoked paprika, chili powder, and dried oregano
- ½ teaspoon salt
- 2 ½ teaspoons cumin, ground
- 15 ounces can diced tomatoes
- 4 garlic cloves, minced
- 1 yellow onion, diced
- For topping; Greek yogurt, cilantro, and green onions

Preparation
- In the slow cooker, add lentils, onion powder, garlic powder, chicken, garlic, onion, cumin, salt, oregano, paprika, chili powder, and chicken broth.
- Cover and cook for 8 hours on low heat.
- Remove chicken into a platter. Cut into small pieces and return into the slow cooker.
- Cook until heated through.
- Top each serving with cilantro, yogurt, and green onions.

Adobo Chicken Soup

Servings: 6

Prep: 15 minutes

Cook: 8 hours

Ingredients
- 1 teaspoon adobo
- 1 pound chicken breast, boneless, skinless
- 1 pound yucca, cubed
- 3 cups chicken broth
- 2 cups water
- 2 tablespoons cilantro
- 1 teaspoon oregano, dried
- 1 tablespoon lime juice
- 1 carrot, chopped
- 1 tablespoon allspice
- 3 garlic cloves
- 2 sticks celery, chopped
- 1 chicken bouillon cube
- ½ cup fideos

Preparation
- Add all ingredients into the slow cooker.
- Cover and cook for 8 hours on low.
- Remove chicken into a plate. Cut into small pieces and return into the slow cooker.
- Mix well and serve.

Thai Chicken Soup

Servings: 4

Prep: 10 minutes

Cook: 10 hours

Ingredients
- 4 chicken thighs, skinless, boneless
- 3 cups chicken stock
- 2 tablespoons fish sauce
- 2 tablespoons soy sauce
- 4 tablespoons red curry paste
- 1 tablespoon palm sugar
- 4 garlic cloves, minced
- 1 ginger piece, minced
- 1 red bell pepper, chopped
- 2 carrots, chopped
- ½ yellow onion, chopped

Preparation

- In the slow cooker, add red bell pepper, yellow onion, carrot, garlic cloves, ginger, fish sauce, soy sauce, red curry paste, palm sugar, chicken and chicken stock.
- Cover and cook for 8 hours on low.
- Transfer chicken into a platter. Cut into small pieces and return into the pot.
- Stir in lime juice. Taste and season as desired
- Serve and enjoy!

Parmesan Chicken Soup

Servings: 4

Prep: 20 minutes

Cook: 4 hours

Ingredients
- ½ cup parmesan cheese, shredded
- ½ pound chicken breast, boneless, skinless, cut into bite size pieces
- 5 cups chicken broth
- 4 ounces penne pasta
- 14.5 ounces crushed tomatoes
- 2 teaspoons oregano, fresh, chopped
- ¼ teaspoon red pepper flakes
- ½ teaspoon black pepper, ground
- 2 tablespoons basil, fresh, chopped
- 1 teaspoon kosher salt
- 2 tablespoons unsalted butter
- 4 garlic cloves, minced
- ½ white onion, chopped
- 1 green bell pepper, chopped

Preparation
- Add all ingredients into the slow cooker except pasta and butter.
- Cover and cook for 3 ½ hours on high.
- Add pasta and continue cooking until pasta is tender.
- Mix in butter, heat through and serve.

Slow Cooker Chicken Broth

Servings: 5

Prep: 15 minutes

Cook: 10 hours

Ingredients
- 2 ½ pounds chicken pieces, bone-in
- 1 tablespoon dried basil
- 2 stalks celery, chopped
- 1 onion, quartered
- 2 carrots, chopped
- 6 cups of water

Preparation
- In the slow cooker, add all ingredients.
- Cover and cook for 10 hours on low.
- Pour broth through a fine sieve into the pan.
- Discard bones and any other food particle on the sieve.
- Let cool and store appropriately.

Chicken Stock

Servings: 6 cups

Prep: 10 minutes

Cook: 8 hours

Ingredients

- Skin and bones from 1 whole chicken
- 2 quarts water
- 4 garlic cloves
- 3 celery ribs
- 5 sprigs thyme, fresh
- 2 carrots, quartered
- ½ bunch parsley leaves, fresh
- 1 tablespoon whole peppercorns

Preparation

- In the slow cooker, add chicken bones and skin, water, carrots, onions, celery, thyme, parsley, garlic, peppercorns, and bay leaves.
- Cover and cook for 8 hours on low.
- Strain soup into a large bowl. Let it cool and store appropriately.

You Can Have Soup Anytime

Nutribullet is changing the way we cook soup. Gone are the days when you had to wait hours for a pot of vegetable or meat soup to simmer. All you have to do today is add ingredients into your machine, screw the blade on the cup, and voila- you have a healthy soup ready to be savored!

Does that sound so easy to be true? Probably yes, but when you experience it for yourself, you'll understand what I am talking about.

I enjoy soup so much to the point that I sometimes make up reasons to have just one more bowl of it. Soup is almost like tea to me, I can have it anytime of the day including early mornings before rushing to the office, who said you can't eat soup anytime you feel like?

If you would like to have soup for breakfast, prepare ingredients the night before. Wash fruits and vegetables and store in the refrigerator. Don't cut the fruits or chop vegetables because they start losing nutrients once they are cut. You'll do the cutting when ready to make the soup in the morning.

There is no doubt Nutribullet makes smooth and nutritious soups. But you want more than just nutrients or smoothness in a bowl of soup. You want something palatable-something that'll tickle your taste buds. And that is what I hope you'll find in this book-healthy but delicious soups you can enjoy with your entire family.

People have discovered health benefits of soups and are therefore incorporating it into their lifestyle. Soup is not only good for warming you up on cold-winter days or giving you comfort when common cold knocks at your door, it's also a rich source of nutrients provided it is made from vegetables and other healthy foods.

Don't just look at soup as an entrée for lunch or dinner, make it one of your favourite foods that you can eat anytime, that is the only way you'll benefit more from it.

The Nutribullet is not a cheap machine, don't let it waste in your cupboard or cabinet, use it daily. Try out as many recipes and before you know it soups will become part of your DNA, and it'll reward you with a healthy happy body, and long life.
Just have fun with your Nutribullet!

Cucumber Soup

Makes 1 serving
　　Ingredients
2 cucumbers, peeled, sliced
½ cup vegetable broth
1 scallion, chopped
½ teaspoon each; salt and freshly ground pepper
1 avocado, peeled, pitted
2 tablespoons fresh lime juice
Preparation
In the Nutribullet, add cucumber, scallion, avocado, lime juice, vegetable broth, salt and pepper. Extract and enjoy!

Broccoli Soup

Makes 2 servings
　　Ingredients
2 bunches broccoli florets, steamed
1 ½ handful cashews, roasted
1 small onion, diced
1 stick celery
1 pinch each; dried rosemary and thyme
1 garlic clove
Salt and freshly ground black pepper, to taste
1 chicken bouillon cube
1 cup skim milk
1 cup almond milk

Preparation

In the Nutribullet, add broccoli, celery, onion, garlic, cashews, thyme, rosemary, chicken bouillon cube, salt and black pepper, skim milk, and almond. Extract and enjoy!

Butternut Squash Sage Soup

Makes 2 servings

Ingredients

1 butternut squash, seeds removed, halved
5 sage leaves
2 cups water
1 garlic clove
¼ cup cashews
1 teaspoon sea salt
1 tablespoon olive oil

Preparation

Preheat your oven to 400^0 F. Sprinkle butternut squash with oil and cook in the preheated oven until tender, approximately 50 minutes. Remove from the oven and let it cool. Transfer roasted squash into your Nutribullet. Add remaining ingredients. Extract and enjoy!

Potato Leek Soup

Makes 2 to 4 servings
　　Ingredients
3 medium chopped sweet potatoes
1 chopped leek
2 cups broccoli florets
3 ½ cups chicken broth
1 tablespoon olive oil
1 tablespoon water
1 chopped onion
1 peeled and chopped apple

Preparation

Add olive oil in a saucepan and heat over medium-high heat. Sauté leek and onions until tender, approximately 4 minutes. Stir often. Add apple, potatoes and chicken broth. Bring the mixture to a boil. Turn heat to a gentle simmer. Let it simmer for 20 minutes or until potatoes soften. Meanwhile, add water and broccoli in a microwave safe bowl and microwave for 1 minute on high. Before you serve the soup, blend in your Nutribullet and return into the saucepan. Add broccoli, mix well and heat through. Enjoy!

Tomato Soup

Makes 2 servings
　　Ingredients
4 large tomatoes, halved
1 pinch each; sea salt and fresh ground black pepper
1 sprig thyme
1 tablespoon superfood spice blend
3 tablespoons olive oil
½ teaspoon parsley, dried
½ small onion
1 ½ cups water

Preparation

Preheat your oven to 350^0 F. Sprinkle tomatoes with olive oil and spread on a baking tray. Season with salt and pepper and place in the preheated oven to cook for 1 hour. Heat little oil in a skillet over medium-high heat. Add onions and sauté for 4 minutes or until browned. In the Nutribullet, add roasted tomatoes, browned onions, parsley, spice blend, thyme, and water. Extract and enjoy!

Rosemary White Bean Soup

Makes 3 servings
    Ingredients
1 tablespoon fresh rosemary
2 cups white beans, cooked
Sea salt and freshly ground black pepper, to taste
1 tablespoon extra-virgin olive oil
2 fresh sage leaves
2 cups vegetable broth

Preparation
In the Nutribullet, add white beans, rosemary, sage leaves, olive oil, sea salt, black pepper, and broth. Extract and enjoy!

Carrot And Beet Soup

Makes 4 servings

Ingredients

4 carrots, chopped

4 small beets

1 cup vegetable broth

1 cup coconut water

1 cup kale

½ teaspoon pepper, ground

1 teaspoon caraway seeds

4 tablespoons tarragon, fresh

½ teaspoon sea salt

2 stalks celery

Preparation

In the Nutribullet, add carrots, beets, celery, kale, caraway seeds, tarragon, sea salt, pepper, broth, and coconut water. Extract and enjoy!

Carrot And Potato

Makes 2 to 4 servings
　　Ingredients
1 small potato, diced
1 pound carrot, diced
1 tablespoon yogurt
2 tablespoons curry powder
2 tablespoons butter
1 dash cayenne pepper
1 onion, chopped
3 cups chicken broth

Preparation

Melt butter in a stock pot over medium heat. Sauté onions until tender, about 5 minutes. Stir from time to time. Stir in carrot, cayenne pepper, curry powder, and chicken broth. Bring the mixture to a boil. Reduce heat to medium-low. Simmer for 20 minutes. Transfer into your Nutribullet and blend until smooth. Top each serving of soup with yogurt.

Tomato And Basil Soup

Makes 1 serving
    Ingredients
3 basil leaves
1 cup chopped tomatoes
1 garlic clove
¼ cup water
¼ cup cream
Preparation
Add all ingredients into your Nutribullet. Extract and enjoy!

Spiced Pumpkin Soup

Makes 2 servings
> Ingredients

1 cup pumpkin puree
2 tablespoons pumpkin seeds
¼ teaspoon nutmeg
½ teaspoon cinnamon
¼ teaspoon fresh pepper
¼ teaspoon salt
2 small beets, chopped
¼ cup chopped onions
1 ½ cups vegetable stock
3 small new potatoes, chopped
½ cup light coconut milk
2 tablespoons olive oil

Preparation

Preheat your oven to 400^0 F. Spread potatoes, onions and beets on a baking tray. Sprinkle with oil and season with salt. Place into the preheated oven and bake until potatoes soften, about 35 minutes. Let it cool and transfer into the Nutribullet. Add all remaining ingredients. Extract and enjoy!

Cherry Tomato Soup

Makes 3 servings

Ingredients

2 cups cherry tomatoes
Freshly squeezed juice from 1 lime
1 pinch each; sea salt and red pepper flakes
½ (13.5 ounces) can coconut milk, full fat
5 basil leaves
1 inch ginger
½ cup cashews

Preparation

In the Nutribullet, add tomatoes, cashews, ginger, basil, sea salt, red pepper flakes, lime juice, and coconut milk. Extract and enjoy!

Tasty Vegetable Soup

Makes 4 servings

Ingredients

½ cup broccoli florets
1 carrot, chopped
2 cups potatoes, peeled, chopped
1 onion, chopped
½ cup cauliflower
1 tablespoon butter
2 tablespoons olive oil
1 pinch cumin
Sea salt and freshly ground black pepper, to taste
Parmesan cheese, for garnish
3 cups vegetable broth

Preparation

Heat oil and butter in a skillet over medium-high heat. Add onions and carrots, cook until tender. Mix in cauliflower, potatoes and broccoli. Add vegetable stock and season to taste with cumin, salt and pepper. Put to simmer for 20 minutes. Remove from heat and allow to cool. Blend in your Nutribullet until smooth. Serve garnished with cheese.

Quick Watermelon Gazpacho

Makes 4 servings

Ingredients

3 cups watermelon

1 tablespoon olive oil

¼ cup fresh lemon juice

Sea salt and black pepper, to taste

2 tablespoons parsley

1 cucumber

1 jalapeno

1 small onion

1 bell pepper

Vegetable broth to max line

Preparation

In the Nutribullet, add watermelon, cucumber, jalapeno, onion, bell pepper, parsley, lemon juice, vegetable broth, olive oil, sea salt, and black pepper. Extract and enjoy!

Cauliflower Soup

Makes 2 serving
   Ingredients
1 head cauliflower
1 cup coconut milk
1 pinch cinnamon
1 teaspoon turmeric powder
½ onion
2 teaspoons extra-virgin olive oil
1 teaspoon cumin
¼ cup cilantro
¼ cup cashews
2 tablespoons curry powder
Sea salt and freshly ground black pepper

Preparation

In the Nutribullet, add cauliflower, cashews, cilantro, cumin, onion, turmeric powder, cinnamon, curry powder, coconut milk, olive oil, sea salt and black pepper. Extract and enjoy!

Pea Soup

Makes 2 servings
  Ingredients
3 cups fresh peas
2 ½ cups vegetable stock
2 shallots, peeled, sliced
Sea salt and black pepper, to taste
½ cup plain Greek yogurt
2 teaspoons olive oil
Tarragon, to taste
Preparation
In the Nutribullet, add peas, shallots, olive oil, yogurt, tarragon, vegetable stock, sea salt, and pepper. Extract and enjoy!

Roasted Carrot Soup

Makes 1 serving
　Ingredients
3 carrots, chopped
1 apple, sliced
¼ teaspoon celery seed
1 ½ cups water
Sea salt and fresh ground pepper, to taste
¼ teaspoon thyme
¼ sweet onion, sliced
1 tablespoon super food spice blend
1 tablespoon olive oil

Preparation

Preheat your oven to 425^0F. Spread carrots, apple, onion, and celery seed on the baking tray. Sprinkle with olive oil and bake in the preheated oven for 30 minutes. Remove from the oven to cool. Transfer into the Nutribullet. Add all remaining ingredients. Extract and enjoy!

Cauliflower Pear Soup

Makes 2 servings

Ingredients

1 pear, peeled, cored
½ head cauliflower, chopped
1 cup plain almond milk, unsweetened
1 tablespoon almond butter
Salt and fresh ground pepper, to taste
1 cup water
1 tablespoon virgin coconut oil, cold-pressed
1 tablespoon superfood spice blend
1 ½ tablespoons Dijon mustard

Preparation

In the Nutribullet, add pear, cauliflower, spice blend, almond butter, coconut oil, water and almond milk. Extract and enjoy!

Celery Soup

Makes 1 serving
　Ingredients
1 ½ cups celery
½ cup water
Sea salt and fresh ground pepper
¼ garlic clove
¼ cup cashews
Preparation
In the Nutribullet, add all ingredients. Extract and enjoy!

Abc Soup

Cooking Time: 50 minutes
Servings: 4-5 persons
　　Ingredients
- 1 packet chicken bones
- 100 grams of chicken breast (diced)
- 1 onion (sliced)
- 2 whole potatos (diced)
- 1 carrot (diced)
- 2000 ml of water
- Pepper
- Salt

Method

1. Add chicken bones, chicken, onions, potatoes and carrots to water and simmer for 50 minutes

2. Add pepper and salt to taste before serving

Abalone And Peas Soup

Cooking Time: 15 minutes
Servings: 4-5 persons
　　Ingredients
- 50 grams of chinese dried mushroom (blanched in hot water till soft)
- 100 grams of fresh garden peas (shelled)
- 1 can of abalone (keep juice in can and dice the abalone)
- 100 grams of chicken (diced)
- 1500 ml of water
- 1 teaspoon light soya sauce
- Salt

Method

1. Add mushrooms, chicken, light soya sauce and salt in water and bring to boil

2. Add peas and abalone juice and boil for another 5 minutes

3. Add abalone and soya sauce and bring to boil

4. Salt to taste and serve

Abalone And Chicken Soup

Cooking Time: 15 minutes
Servings: 4-5 persons
   Ingredients
- 1 can of abalone (keep juice in can and slice the abalone)
- 100 grams of chicken (diced)
- 1 tablespoon of chinese wine
- 1000 ml of water
- 1 tablespoon corn flour
- 1 teaspoon light soya sauce
- Salt

Method

1. Mix well cornflour, soya sauce, chinese wine and salt with chicken.

2. Add water and abalone juice and bring to boil

3. Add marinated chicken and bring to boil for further 5 minutes

4. Add abalone and bring to boil

5. Salt to taste and serve

Asparagus Soup

Cooking Time: 50 minutes
Servings: 4-6 persons
   Ingredients
- 100 grams of chicken breast (diced)
- 1000 ml of water
- Small Bundle of Fresh Asapargus (diagionally sliced 1 inch long)
- Ginger (thinly sliced)
- 1 teaspoon cornflour
- 2-3 tablespoon cold water
- Salt

Method

1. Put chicken, ginger and asparagus in water and bring to boil

2. Simmer for 45 minutes

4. Thicken with cornflour and cold water, slowly add in while stirring

5. Add salt to taste and serve

Bean Sprouts And Egg Drop Soup

Cooking Time: 15 minutes
Servings: 4 persons
   Ingredients
- 100 grams of bean sprouts (washed)
- 100 grams of chicken (diced)
- 2 eggs, well beaten
- 1500 ml of water
- 1 teaspoon light soya sauce
- Salt
Method

1. Add chicken to water and bring to boil, simmer for 8 minutes

2. Add bean sprouts and light soya sauce and simmer for another 5 minutes

3. Stir the soup in a circular motion and pour the egg at the same time.

4. Salt to taste and serve

Bird's Nest Soup

Cooking Time: 9 hours 20 minutes
Servings: 4 persons
  Ingredients
- 100 grams of birds nest (soaked in hot water for 4 hours)
- 1 chicken leg (with skin)
- 1 pack of chicken bones
- 2 teaspoons of water chestnut flour
- 2 tablespoon cold water
- 2000 ml of water
- 1 egg white
- Pepper
- Salt

Method

1. Simmer chicken bones with water for 2 hours.

2. Add broth to bird's nest and chicken leg and steam for 3 hours

3. Remove chicken leg and allow to cool, slowly peel into strips

4. Place bird's nest and broth into saucepan and bring to boil

5. Mix water chestnut flour and cold water

6. Season with salt and pepper and stirring in water chestnut mix

7. Simmer for 2 minutes, stirring all the time

8. Add in white of egg and salt to taste

9. Add in chicken shreds and serve.

Cabbage And Prawn Soup

Cooking Time: 20 minutes
Servings: 4-5 persons
    Ingredients
- 100 grams of fresh prawns (shelled)
- 2-3 Chinese cabbage heads (shredded)
- 1500 ml of water
- Ginger (thinly sliced)
- 1 teaspoon light soya sauce
- 2 tablespoon cornflour
- 2-3 tablespoon of cold water
- Salt

Method

1. Put salt, ginger and cabbage in water and bring to boil for 8 minutes

2. Mix cornflour with water and slowly pour into soup while stirring

3. Bring to boil and add in prawns and light soya sauce

4. Salt to taste and serve

Tip: To maintain cabbage colour, keep the pot uncovered while simmering

Cabbage Soup

Cooking Time: 20 minutes
Servings: 4-5 persons
   Ingredients
- 80 grams of pork (diced)
- 2-3 Chinese cabbage heads (shredded)
- 1500 ml of water
- Ginger (thinly sliced)
- 1 teaspoon light soya sauce
- Salt

Method

1. Boil pork and ginger in water for 15 minutes.

2. Add in light soya sauce and cabbage and simmer for further 5 minutes

3. Add salt to taste and serve

Tip: To maintain cabbage colour, keep the pot uncovered while simmering

Celery Soup

Cooking Time: 10 minutes (1 day marinating needed)
Servings: 4-5 persons

Ingredients

- 2 tablespoon of canola oil
- 150 grams of beef (diced)
- Small bundle of celery (diagionally sliced 1-inch)
- 1500 ml of water
- Ginger (thinly sliced)
- 1 teaspoon light soya sauce
- 1 teaspoon of white pepper
- 1 teaspoon of sesame oil
- Salt

Method

1. Mix the oil, soya sauce, salt and pepper to form a marinate

2. Pour marinate onto beef, mix evenly and place in fridge for at least a day

3. Put celery and ginger into water and bring to boil

4. Add sesame oil and marinated beef and bring to boil

5. Salt to taste and serve

Chicken And Sweet Corn Soup

Cooking Time: 55 minutes
Servings: 4-6 persons

Ingredients

- 100 grams of chicken breast (diced)
- 150 grams of chicken bones (washed)
- 1000 ml of water
- 200 grams of sweet corn
- 1 egg, well-beaten
- 1 teaspoon cornflour
- 2-3 tablespoon of cold water
- Ginger (thinly sliced)
- Salt

Method

1. Bring to boil a pot of water, chicken bones and ginger.

2. Add the diced chicken into the pot, bring to boil and simmer for 45 minutes.

3. Proceed by adding the sweet corn and further simmer for 5 minutes

4. Stir the soup in a circular motion and pour the egg at the same time. This would create egg shreds.

5. Season to taste.

6. Before serving, further thicken with cornflour and water

Chicken And Ham Soup

Cooking Time: 3 hours 10 minutes
Servings: 4 persons
　　Ingredients
- 1 whole chicken (small, cleaned)
- 4000 ml of water
- 100 grams of prawns (shelled)
- 2 tablespoon of chinese wine
- 100 grams of chinese ham (shredded)
- Pepper
- Salt

Method

1. Put chicken in water and bring to boil

2. Add in prawns, chinese wine, pepper, salt and ham

3. Simmer gently for 3 hours

4. Salt to taste and serve

Chicken And Mushroom Soup

Cooking Time: 10 minutes
Servings: 4 persons
    Ingredients
- 100 grams of chicken breast (diced)
- 1500 ml of water
- 100 grams of mushroom (sliced)
- 100 grams of bamboo shoots (sliced)
- 2 tablespoon of chinese wine
- 1 teaspoon corn flour
- 2 tablespoon cold water
- 1 teaspoon of light soya sauce
- Pepper
- Salt

Method

1. Put chicken in water and bring to boil, simmer for 5 minutes

2. Add mushrooms, bamboo shoots, chinese wine and light soya sauce

3. Mix corn flour with cold water and stir in soup, bring to boil

4. Salt to taste and serve

Chicken Chowder

Cooking Time: 2 hours and 45 minutes
Servings: 6 persons
　　Ingredients
- 1 young chicken (small, cleaned)
- 2 cup of white rice
- 1 packet rice noodles
- 2 teaspoon of canola oil
- Ginger (thinly sliced)
- 1 tablespoon of seasame oil
- 1 tablespoon of light soya sauce
- 4000 ml of water
- Pepper
- Salt

Method

1. Place chicken, ginger, water and rice into water and cook for 2 1/2 hours

2. Aside, heat some oil and cook noodles for 2 minutes. Remove and drain

3. Remove chicken and allow to cool before cutting up into pieces

4. Add chicken back to chowder and cook for further 10 minutes

5. Add sesame oil, salt and pepper to taste

6. Portion out rice noodles and add chowder to cover to serve.

Chicken Soup With Egg

Cooking Time: 2 hours 10 minutes
Servings: 4 persons
　　Ingredients
- 150 grams chicken breast (diced)
- 2 tablespoon corn flour
- 2 table spoon cold water
- 1 teaspoon sugar
- 2000 ml of water
- 1 packet of chicken bones
- 1 teaspoon of sesame oil
- 2 eggs, well beaten
- Pepper
- Salt

Method

1. Simmer chicken bones with 2000ml water for 2 hours.

2. Mix corn flour, water, sugar, salt and pepper and add to broth

3. Add in diced chicken and bring to boil

4. Stir the soup in a circular motion and pour the egg at the same time.

5. Salt to taste and serve

Chicken Soup With Fried Noodles

Cooking Time: 2 hours 10 minutes
Servings: 4 persons
    Ingredients
- 150 grams chicken breast (diced)
- 100 grams of mushrooms (sliced)
- 100 grams of bamboo shoots (sliced)
- 1 round fried noodles
- 2000 ml of water
- 1000 ml of water
- 1 packet of chicken bones
- 1 teaspoon of sesame oil
- Pepper
- Salt

Method

1. Cook noodles with 1000ml of water, drain and put in serving bowl

2. Simmer chicken bones with 2000ml water for 2 hours.

3. Add chicken, mushrooms and bamboo shoots to broth

4. Cover and bring to boil for 3 minutes

5. Add salt and pepper to taste

6. Add sesame oil to serving bowl of noodles

7. Pour broth over noodles and serve

Crab Meat Soup

Cooking Time: 20 minutes
Servings: 4 persons

Ingredients

- 1 large crab or 200 grams of crab meat
- 2 teaspoon of canola oil
- Ginger (thinly sliced)
- 2 tablespoon of chinese wine
- 1 tablespoon of light soya sauce
- 2 cloves garlic crushed
- 2000 ml of water
- 1 egg well beaten
- 1 teaspoon of corn flour
- 2 tablespoon of cold water
- Pepper
- Salt

Method

1. Remove flesh from crab (if using whole crab)

2. Put oil, ginger, chinese wine and light soya sauce into water and bring to boil

3. Add crab meat and simmer for further 10 minutes

4. Mix corn flour with water and stir in slowly

5. Pour egg into soup and stir

6. Season with salt and pepper to taste and serve

Cucumber And Minced Chicken Soup

Cooking Time: 45 minutes
Servings: 6 persons
　　Ingredients
- 100 grams of minced chicken
- 1 cucumber (sliced thinly)
- 1 tablespoon of sesame oil
- 1 tablespoon of light soya sauce
- 1 teaspoon corn flour
- 2000 ml of water
- Pepper
- Salt

Method

1. Mix minced chicken, corn flour, sesame oil and light soya sauce

2. Add sliced cucumbers to water and bring to boil

3. Using a teaspoon, scoop meat mix and drop into water, forming small balls

4. Simmer for 40 minutes

5. Add salt and pepper to taste before serving

Duck And Orange Peel Soup

Cooking Time: 2 hours and 10 minutes
Servings: 6 persons

Ingredients

- 1 young duck (small, cleaned)
- 1 teaspoon of canola oil
- 100 grams dried orange peel
- 1 packet of chicken bones
- 4000 ml of water
- Pepper
- Salt

Method

1. Simmer chicken bones in water for 1 hour

2. Aside, heat oil and brown duck on all sides.

3. Take duck out, drain, allow to cool before cutting into pieces

4. Using the same oil, heat orange peel slightly and put into broth

5. After cutting the duck, add duck into broth and continue to boil for another hour

6. Add salt and pepper to taste before serving

Duck And Salted Vegetable Soup

Cooking Time: 2 hours and 10 minutes
Servings: 6 persons
　　Ingredients
- 1 young duck (small, cleaned)
- 1 teaspoon of canola oil
- 200 grams salted vegetables (sliced)
- 4000 ml of water
- Pepper
- Salt

Method

1. Add salted vegetables to water and simmer for 1 hour

2. Aside, heat oil and brown duck on all sides.

3. Take duck out, drain, allow to cool before cutting into pieces

4. After cutting the duck, add duck into broth and continue to boil for another hour

6. Add salt and pepper to taste before serving

Egg Soup

Cooking Time: 15 minutes
Servings: 4-5 persons
　　Ingredients
- 1/2 teaspoon of canola oil
- 1000 ml of water
- 80 grams of pork (shredded)
- 2 eggs, well beaten
- 1 teaspoon light soya sauce
- Salt

Method

1. Heat oil in sauce pan, add pork and stir till fragrant.

2. Add water and bring to boil

3. Add salt to taste and simmer for 5 minutes.

4. Add eggs, season with soya sauce and serve.

Fish Chowder

Cooking Time: 2 hours and 45 minutes
Servings: 6 persons

Ingredients

- 200 grams of fish fillet (thinly sliced)
- 2 cup of white rice
- 100 grams dried mushroom (sliced)
- 1 packet rice noodles
- 2 teaspoon of canola oil
- Ginger (thinly sliced)
- 1 tablespoon of sesame oil
- 1 tablespoon of light soya sauce
- 4000 ml of water
- 1 egg well beaten
- Pepper
- Salt

Method

1. Heat some oil and cook noodles for 2 minutes. Remove and drain

2. Mix corn flour with water and coat with sliced fish fillet

3. Add ginger, sesame oil, light soya sauce, mushroom, rice in water and cook for 2 hours

4. Add in fish fillet and egg, cook for 2-3 minutes

5. Add sesame oil, salt and pepper to taste

6. Portion out rice noodles and add chowder to cover to serve.

Fish Soup

Cooking Time: 45 minutes
Servings: 6 persons
    Ingredients
- 500 grams of fish fillet (thinly sliced)
- 200 grams of dried silver fish
- 2 teaspoon of chinese wine
- Ginger (thinly sliced)
- 1 tablespoon of sesame oil
- 1 tofu (diced)
- 1 tablespoon of light soya sauce
- 3000 ml of water
- 1 egg well beaten
- 1 tomato (cut into half)
- Pepper
- Salt

Method

1. Add dried silver fish, tomatoes and ginger to water and simmer for 30 minutes

2. Add in chinese wine, sesame oil, light soya sauce, tofu and fish and simmer for 10 minutes

3. Stir the soup in a circular motion and pour the egg at the same time

4. Season to taste before serve

Lettuce And Egg Drop Soup

Cooking Time: 45 minutes
Servings: 4-5 persons
　　Ingredients
- 150 grams of pork (diced)
- 1 small lettuce (shredded)
- 1500 ml of water
- Ginger (thinly sliced)
- 2 eggs, well beaten
- 1 teaspoon light soya sauce
- Salt

Method

1. Boil pork and ginger in water for 30 minutes.

2. Add in light soya sauce and lettuce and bring to boil

3. Stir the soup in a circular motion and pour the egg at the same time.

4. Add salt to taste and serve

Lettuce And Shrimp Soup

Cooking Time: 20 minutes
Servings: 4-5 persons

Ingredients
- 80 grams of pork (diced)
- 1 small lettuce (shredded)
- 20 grams of dried shrimps (washed and dried)
- 1500 ml of water
- Ginger (thinly sliced)
- 1 teaspoon light soya sauce
- Salt

Method

1. Boil pork, shrimps and ginger in water for 15 minutes.

2. Add in light soya sauce and lettuce and bring to boil

3. Add salt to taste and serve

Mixed Vegetables Soup

Cooking Time: 30 minutes
Servings: 4 persons
　　Ingredients
- 100 grams of fresh mushrooms (sliced)
- 1 bunch of spinach (washed)
- 1 small bunch of water cress (washed)
- 1000 ml of water
- 1 teaspoon light soya sauce
- 2 tablespoon sesame oil
- 1 teaspoon of white pepper
- Salt

Method

1. Stir fry fresh mushrooms in sesame oil for 5 minutes

2. Add salt, pepper and light soya sauce in water and bring to boil

3. Add fried mushrooms and bring to boil

4. Add spinach and water cress and bring to boil

5. Salt to taste and serve

Mushroom And Peas Soup

Cooking Time: 20 minutes
Servings: 4-5 persons
　　　Ingredients
- 100 grams of chinese dried mushroom (blanched in hot water till soft)
- 100 grams of fresh garden peas (shelled)
- 100 grams of chicken (diced)
- 1500 ml of water
- Ginger (thinly sliced)
- 1 teaspoon of white pepper
- 1 teaspoon light soya sauce
- Salt

Method

1. Add mushrooms, ginger, white pepper, light soya sauce and salt in water and bring to boil

2. Add in chicken and peas and simmer for 15 minutes uncovered

3. Salt to taste and serve

Mushroom Soup

Cooking Time: 50 minutes
Servings: 4-5 persons
    Ingredients
- 150 grams of chinese dried mushroom (blanched in hot water till soft)
- 200 grams of beef (diced)
- 3000 ml of water
- Ginger (thinly sliced)
- 1 egg (well beaten)
- 1 teaspoon of white pepper
- Salt

Method

1. Add mushrooms, beef, white pepper and ginger into water and bring to boil

2. Simmer for 45 minutes

3. Add egg slowly to form strips

4. Salt to taste and serve

Prawn Soup Rice

Cooking Time: 35 minutes
Servings: 4-6 persons
   Ingredients
- 300 grams of raw prawns (peeled, heads separated)
- 1 cup of white rice (washed)
- 1000 ml of water
- Ginger (thinly sliced)
- 1 packet of Bak Choy (4-5 stalks, washed)
- Dark Soya Sauce (to add colour and a bit of soy taste)
- Salt

Method

1. Bring to boil a pot of water with the raw prawn heads, ginger and peels and simmer for 30 minutes.

2. Remove the prawn peels leaving the head and add the washed white rice.

3. Simmer until the rice softens which would result in a thicken soup

4. Add the prawns and bak choy and simmer for 5 minutes

5. Season to taste with salt and dark soya sauce (only a bit) before serve

Peas And Egg Drop Soup

Cooking Time: 30 minutes
Servings: 4-5 persons
    Ingredients
- 100 grams of chicken breast (diced)
- 1250 ml of water
- 100 grams of young green peas
- Ginger (thinly sliced)
- 2 eggs, well beaten
- 1 teaspoon light soya sauce
- Salt

Method

1. Put chicken, ginger and peas in water and bring to boil

2. Simmer for 30 minutes and add light soya sauce

3. Stir the soup in a circular motion and pour the egg at the same time.

4. Add salt to taste and serve

Pigeon Soup

Cooking Time: 1 hour
Servings: 6 persons
   Ingredients
- 2 young pigeons (cleaned and cut into quarters)
- 100 grams dried mushroom (soaked and sliced)
- 2 teaspoon of chinese wine
- 1 tablespoon of light soya sauce
- 2000 ml of water
- Pepper
- Salt

Method

1. Place all ingredients into saucepan and bring to boil
2. Simmer for 50 minutes
3. Season to taste and serve

Roast Pork And Mushroom Soup

Cooking Time: 15 minutes
Servings: 4 persons
　　Ingredients
- 100 grams of chinese roast pork (sliced)
- 1500 ml of water
- 100 grams of mushroom (sliced)
- 100 grams of bamboo shoots (sliced)
- 2 tablespoon of chinese wine
- 1 teaspoon corn flour
- 2 tablespoon cold water
- 1 teaspoon of light soya sauce
- Pepper
- Salt

Method

1. Put roast pork in water and bring to boil, simmer for 5 minutes

2. Add mushrooms, bamboo shoots, chinese wine and light soya sauce

3. Mix corn flour with cold water and stir in soup, bring to boil

4. Salt to taste and serve

Shark's Fin Soup

Cooking Time: 6 hours and 20 minutes (1 day preparation)
Servings: 6 persons

Ingredients
- 500 grams of shark fin
- Ginger (thinly sliced)
- 2 cloves of garlic (crushed)
- 1 packet of chicken bones
- 100 grams of chicken breast
- 4000 ml of water
- 100 grams bamboo shoots (sliced)
- 1 egg well beaten
- 2 teaspoon of corn flour
- 2 tablespoon of cold water
- 1 tablespoon soya sauce
- Pepper
- Salt

Method

1. Soak shark fins in water for 24 hours

2. Boil shark fins in water with ginger and garlic for 4 hours

3. Drain and remove any flesh on the fins

4. Aside, cook chicken bones and chicken leg in water and simmer for 4 hours

5. Remove chicken leg and shred

6. Put shark fins, bamboo shoot and shredded chicken into broth and boil for 10 minutes

7. Stir the soup in a circular motion and pour the egg at the same time

8 Mix corn flour with cold water and stir in slowly to thicken the soup

9. Add soya sauce, salt and pepper to taste before serve.

Spinach Soup

Cooking Time: 15 minutes
Servings: 4 persons
　　Ingredients
- 1 bundle of spinach (washed)
- 100 grams of chicken (diced)
- 1500 ml of water
- 1 teaspoon light soya sauce
- Salt

Method

1. Add chicken in water and bring to boil

2. Add spinach, salt and soya sauce and simmer on low heat for 5 minutes

3. Salt to taste and serve

Sweet Corn With Pork And Egg Shreds Soup

Cooking Time: 55 minutes
Servings: 4-6 persons

Ingredients

- 500 grams of lean pork (diced)
- 1000 ml of water
- 200 grams of sweet corn
- 1 egg, well-beaten
- 1 teaspoon cornflour
- 2-3 tablespoon of cold water
- Ginger (thinly sliced)
- Salt

Method

1. Bring to boil a pot of water and ginger.

2. Add the diced pork into the pot, bring to boil and simmer for 45 minutes.

3. Proceed by adding the sweet corn and further simmer for 5 minutes

4. Stir the soup in a circular motion and pour the egg at the same time. This would create egg shreds.

5. Season to taste.

6. Before serving, further thicken with cornflour and water

Tomato And Egg Soup

Cooking Time: 25 minutes
Servings: 4 persons
　　Ingredients
- 100 grams of tomatoes (chopped and peeled)
- 100 grams of chicken (diced)
- 1500 ml of water
- 2 tablespoon cold water
- 1 teaspoon sugar
- 1 teaspoon light soya sauce
- 1 teaspoon white pepper
- 2 eggs, well beaten
- Salt

Method

1. Add chicken and tomatoes in water and bring to boil for 20 minutes

2. Mix well cornflour, water, sugar, salt and pepper, add mixture to soup

3. Stir the soup in a circular motion and pour the egg at the same time.

4. Salt to taste and serve

Wan Ton Soup

Cooking Time: 45 minutes
Servings: 6 persons
 Ingredients
- 100 grams of minced pork
- 100 grams of prawns (shelled and minced)
- 1 packet of wan ton skin
- 1 teaspoon of corn flour
- 1 teaspoon of chinese wine
- 1 teaspoon of canola oil
- 1 tablespoon of sesame oil
- 1 tablespoon of light soya sauce
- 3000 ml of water
- 1 egg well beaten
- 1 egg white
- Pepper
- Salt

Method

1. Add minced prawn, pork, corn flour, chinese wine, canola oil, sesame oil, light soya sauce, beaten egg into bowl and mix well

2. Using a teaspoon, scoop some mix and place it in center of wan ton skin

3. Using your fingers, dap some egg white along the sides of the wan ton skin (without touching the meat mix) before folding it together

4. Once all wan ton is done, boil water

5. Add wan ton into boiling water and cook covered for 5 minutes

6. Add salt and pepper to taste and serve

Watercress Soup

Cooking Time: 10 minutes
Servings: 4 persons
    Ingredients
- 1 bunch of watercress (washed)
- 100 grams of chicken (diced)
- 1500 ml of water
- Ginger (thinly sliced)
- 2 pieces dried tangerine peel
- 1 teaspoon light soya sauce
- Salt

Method

1. Add chicken, tangerine peel and ginger in water, bring to boil, simmer for 7 minutes

2. Add watercress and light soya sauce and bring to boil

3. Salt to taste and serve

Whole Chicken With Bird's Nest Soup

Cooking Time: 3 hours 20 minutes
Servings: 6 persons
   Ingredients
- 100 grams of birds nest (soaked in hot water for 4 hours)
- 1 chicken whole (small - cleaned)
- 1 chicken leg (with skin)
- 3 teaspoons of chinese wine
- 1 pack of chicken bones
- 2000 ml of water
- Pepper
- Salt

Method

1. Simmer chicken bones with water for 2 hours.

2. Add broth to bird's nest and chicken leg and steam for 3 hours

3. Remove chicken leg and allow to cool, slowly peel into strips

4. Place bird's nest and broth into saucepan and bring to boil

5. Add pepper and salt to taste

6. Add in chinese wine and chicken shreds

7. Wrap whole chicken in aluminium foil, leaving the top open

8. Pour in bird's nest broth and cover aluminium foil (careful its hot)

9. Steam for 1 hour

10. Put whole chicken in aluminium foil in big bowl before opening to serve

Creamy Spinach Soup

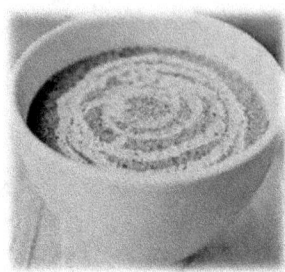

The adorable, leafy spinach in this recipe makes for a flavorsome and fascinating vivid-green soup

- Ready: 1¼ hrs.
- Serves: 4 servings

INGREDIENTS
- ☐ 50g butter
- ☐ 1 medium onion, finely chopped
- ☐ 2 garlic cloves, finely chopped
- ☐ 1 medium potato, peeled and chopped into chunks
- ☐ 450ml chicken or vegetable stock
- ☐ 600ml milk
- ☐ 450g fresh spinach, washed if necessary and roughly chopped
- ☐ finely grated zest of half a lemon
- ☐ freshly grated nutmeg, to taste
- ☐ 3 tablespoons double cream, to serve

DIRECTIONS
1. Melt the butter in a big lidded saucepan, add the onion and garlic and fry gently for five-6 mins until softening. Stir in the potato and retain to prepare dinner lightly for 1 minute. Pour inside the stock and simmer for eight-10 mins until the potato starts off evolved to cook. Pour inside the milk and

bring as much as a simmer, then stir in half of the spinach and the lemon zest. Cowl and simmer for 15 mins until the spinach has completely wilted down. Allow to chill for approximately five mins.

2. Pour the soup into a blender (ideally) or food processor, upload the final spinach (this could keep the soup bright inexperienced and sparkling tasting) and procedure until silky clean – you could want to do this in batches depending on the dimensions of your machine. (The soup might also now be frozen for up to at least one month. Defrost within the microwave or overnight inside the fridge. The soup may additionally lose a number of its vibrancy on freezing, but the flavor won't be impaired.) Return to the pan and reheat. Taste and season with salt, pepper and nutmeg. You may like to dilute the soup with a touch extra inventory if too thick. Ladle the soup into bowls and swirl within the cream

TIP
Getting it bright green

The secret of a fresh-flavored, shiny green soup is to cook dinner half of the spinach in short inside the soup for intensity of flavor, then add the final raw spinach while liquidizing.

Pumpkin Soup

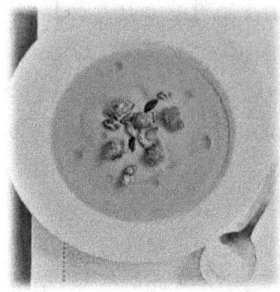

A silky textured soup, sprinkled via crunchy croutons & seeds
- Preparation: 20 minutes
- Cook: 25 minutes
- Serves: 6 servings

INGREDIENTS
- ☐ 4 tablespoons olive oil
- ☐ 2 onions, finely chopped
- ☐ 1kg pumpkins or squash (try kabocha), peeled, deseeded and chopped into chunks
- ☐ 700ml vegetable stock or chicken stock
- ☐ 142ml pot double cream
- ☐ 4 slices whole meal seeded bread
- ☐ handful pumpkin seed from a packet

DIRECTIONS
1. Preheat 2 tablespoons olive oil in a big saucepan, then lightly prepare dinner 2 finely chopped onions for five minutes, till soft but now not colored. Upload 1kg peeled, deseeded and chopped pumpkin or squash to the pan, then keep on cooking for 8-10 minutes, stirring every now and then till it starts off evolved to melt and flip golden.

2. Pour 700ml vegetable stock into the pan, then season with salt and pepper. Convey to the boil, and then simmer for 10 minutes until the squash is very gentle. Pour the 142ml pot of double cream into the pan; bring again to the boil, then purée with a hand blender. For an extra-velvety consistency you may now push the soup thru a fine sieve into every other pan. The soup can now be frozen for up to 2 months.

3. Whilst the soup is cooking, slice the crusts from 4 slices of whole meal seed bread, then reduce the bread into small croutons. Warmness the closing 2 tablespoons olive oil in a frying pan, then fry the bread until it begins to emerge as crisp. Add a handful of pumpkin seeds to the pan, and then cook dinner for a few mins extra till they're toasted. Those may be made an afternoon ahead and stored in an airtight container. Reheat the soup if needed, flavor for seasoning, then serve scattered with croutons and seeds and drizzled with more olive oil, if you need.

TIP
Or why no longer try...

Taking the tops off entire acorn squash, scooping out seeds and roasting entire till tender. Stuff with goat's cheese and basil, then cook until the cheese has melted.

Cream Of Wild Mushroom Soup

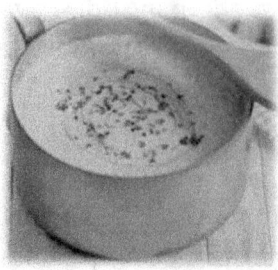

This rich and filling dish is the appropriate manner to dissipate gives up-of-season mushrooms on the cheap

- Preparation: 30 minutes
- Cook: 40 minutes
- Serves: 4 servings

INGREDIENTS
- ☐ 25g dried porcini (ceps)
- ☐ 50g butter
- ☐ 1 onion, finely chopped
- ☐ 1 garlic clove, sliced
- ☐ thyme sprigs
- ☐ 400g blended wild mushrooms
- ☐ 850ml vegetable stock
- ☐ 200ml tub crème fraiche
- ☐ 4 slices white bread, about 100g, cubed
- ☐ chives and truffle oil, to serve

DIRECTIONS
1. Convey a kettle to the boil, and then pour the water over the dried porcini just to cover. Warmth half the butter in a saucepan, then lightly sizzle the onion, garlic and thyme for 5 minutes until softened and beginning to brown. Drain the porcini, booking the juice, then upload to the onion with the

blended wild mushrooms. Leave to cook for 5 minutes until they cross limp. Pour over the stock and the reserved juices, convey to the boil, and then simmer for 20 minutes. Stir in crème fraiche, and then simmer for some minutes more. Blitz the soup with a hand blender or liquidizer, bypass through a first-rate sieve, and then set aside.

2. Preheat the last butter in a frying pan, fry the bread cubes till golden, then drain on kitchen paper. To serve, preheat the soup and froth up with a hand blender, if you like. Ladle the soup into bowls, scatter over the croutons and chives and drizzle via truffle oil.

TIP
Why no longer try?

Combined wild mushrooms are scrumptious pro and fried in olive oil or butter, then piled onto buttered toast and topped with a poached egg.

Spinach Soup

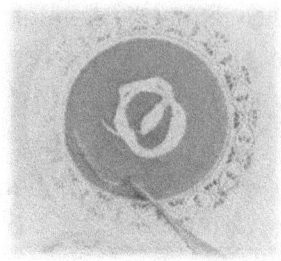

A vibrant green combined soup with half of-fats crème fraiche it truly is healthy and filling - make a batch and freeze

- Preparation: 10 minutes
- Cook: 25 minutes
- Serves: 4 servings

INGREDIENTS

☐ 25g butter
☐ 1 bunch spring onions, chopped
☐ 1 leek (approximately 120g), sliced
☐ 2 small sticks celery (approximately 85g), sliced
☐ 1 small potato (approximately 200g), peeled and diced
☐ ½ tsp ground black pepper
☐ 1l stock (made with 2 chicken or vegetable stock cubes)
☐ 2 x 200-235g bags spinach
☐ 150g half-fat crème fraiche

DIRECTIONS

1. Preheat the butter in a big saucepan. Upload; the spring onions, leek, celery and potato. Stir and put on the lid. Sweat for 10 mins, stirring multiple times.
2. Pour within the stock and cook for 10 – 15 mins till the potato is soft.

3. Upload the spinach and cook for a couple of mins till wilted. Use a hand blender to blitz to a smooth soup.
4. Stir in the crème fraiche. Heat and serve.

TIP
Dinner party trick

Drizzle with double cream for a colorful contrast that looks terrific in your dinner party desk.

Shirred Squash Soup

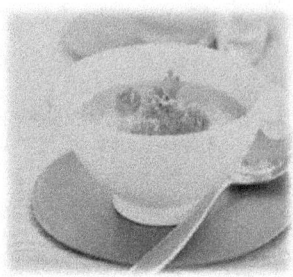

A very good soup quickly will become a failsafe recipe for any event. You can always pass over out the sherry if making for youngsters

- Preparation: 20 minutes
- Cook: 30 minutes
- Serves: 4 servings

INGREDIENTS
- ☐ 1 big onion, halved
- ☐ 4 tablespoons dry (fino) sherry
- ☐ 1kg butternut squash peeled, deseeded and chopped
- ☐ 600ml hot vegetable stock (we like Marigold)
- ☐ seed bread croutons and flat leaf parsley
- ☐ 2 tablespoons olive oil

DIRECTIONS
1. Fry the onion in the oil for 5 minutes till softened. Upload the sherry and squash and sizzle for 1-2 minutes. Pour inside the inventory, then cowl and simmer for 20 minutes till the squash is soft whilst pierced with a knife.
2. Whizz in a meals processor until soft. Will hold in the fridge for 2 days, or freeze for 6 weeks. When ready to devour, preheat until bubbling and serve in small quantities topped

with seed-bread croutons (see above right) and a parsley sprig.

Frothy Cannellini Soup

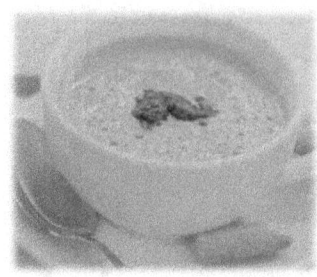

Lesley Waters' impressive soup makes a fashionable, frothy and smooth starter - strive serving in a cappuccino cup

- Ready: 30 mins
- Serves: 8 servings

INGREDIENTS
- ☐ 3 tablespoons olive oil
- ☐ 1 large onion, finely chopped
- ☐ 2 garlic cloves, crushed
- ☐ 1 medium leek, thinly sliced
- ☐ 3 sticks celery, finely chopped
- ☐ 400g cans cannellini beans, drained and rinsed
- ☐ 1.7l vegetable stock
- ☐ 1 bay leaf
- ☐ 142ml carton double cream
- ☐ 150g pot fresh green pesto from the chiller cabinet
- ☐ 125g pack (around 16) sesame breadsticks, optional

DIRECTIONS
1. Preheat the oil in a big saucepan and tip within the onion, garlic, leek and celery. Cover and sweat the vegetables over low warmth for eight-10 minutes till softened.
2. Upload the beans, stock and bay leaf, then season and produce to the boil. Decrease the warmth, then simmer,

covered, for 20-25 minutes till the veggies is completely softened. Permit to chill barely.

3. Whizz via a stick blender until soft, pour inside the cream and preheat. The soup may be refrigerated or frozen at this point.

4. Earlier than serving, upload half the pesto and whizz once more for only some seconds until the soup is flecked with basil. Season to taste. Ladle the soup into 8 cappuccino cups or bowls and spoon a dollop of the last pesto into each serving.

TIP
The usage of a frother

When you have a cappuccino frother, you could use it to give eating place-style frothiness to the soup. Whizz each serving for some seconds, in the cup.

Simple Coconut & Bean Soup

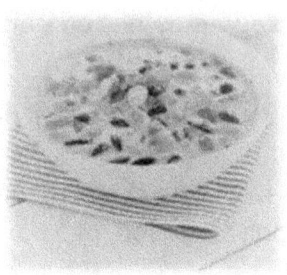

This vegetarian meal in a bowl shows how something yummy may be made from broadly speaking store cupboard ingredients

- Preparation: 10 minutes
- Cook: 20 minutes
- Serves: 4 servings

INGREDIENTS

☐ 1 tablespoons sunflower oil
☐ ½ bunch spring onions, whites and greens separated and sliced
☐ 1 red pepper, diced
☐ 1 Scotch bonnet chili, deseeded and pounded to a paste
☐ 1 garlic clove, chopped
☐ 1 teaspoon dried thyme
☐ 1 teaspoon medium curry powder
☐ 1 teaspoon allspice
☐ 3 plum tomatoes, chopped
☐ 1 vegetable stock cube
☐ 410g can kidney beans, rinsed and drained
☐ 410g can pinto beans, rinsed and drained
☐ 410g can black-eyed beans, rinsed and drained
☐ 2 x 400g cans coconut milk
☐ juice 2 limes

DIRECTIONS
1. Preheat the oil in a big saucepan. Sizzle the spring onion whites, pepper, chili paste and garlic for five-8 minutes till soft and fragrant. Upload the thyme, curry powder and spices, then cook dinner for 1 minute more, Stir in the tomatoes, then prepare dinner for two minutes to soften barely.
2. Disintegrate within the stock cube, and then tip in all the beans and the coconut milk. Simmer for 10 minutes. Flip off the heat and stir in maximum of the spring onion vegetables, the lime juice and some seasoning. Ladle into bowls and scatter with residual spring onions just earlier than serving.

Lightly Spiced Carrot Soup

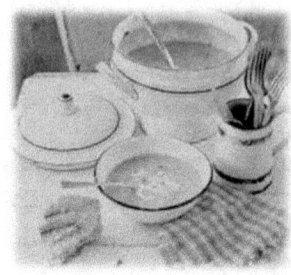

A fulfilling soup which is delicately spiced and works properly as a rustic starter

- Preparation: 10 minutes
- Cook: 25 minutes
- Serves: 6 servings

INGREDIENTS

- ☐ 1 tablespoon vegetable oil
- ☐ 1 onion, finely chopped
- ☐ 1 garlic clove, chopped
- ☐ knob of fresh root ginger, grated
- ☐ 1 red chili, deseeded and chopped
- ☐ 1 teaspoon mild curry powder, plus extra
- ☐ 1kg carrots, trimmed and sliced
- ☐ 2 lemongrass stalks, bashed
- ☐ 2 strips orange zest
- ☐ 400g can coconut milk
- ☐ 700ml vegetable stock

DIRECTIONS

1. Preheat the oil in a huge pan with a lid. Tip inside the onion, garlic, ginger and chili, then cook dinner for three-five minutes until smooth. Stir in the curry powder, accompanied

by means of the carrots, lemongrass and zest, then cover and prepare dinner over a low heat for 10 minutes extra.

2. Deliver the coconut milk can a shake, and then pour most of it into the pan along with the vegetable inventory. Deliver to the boil, then turn down and simmer for 15 minutes till the carrots are really smooth. Do away with the lemongrass and orange zest, and then use a stick blender or food processor to whizz till soft. Ladle into bowls and top with a swirl of reserved coconut milk and an extra sprinkling of curry powder, if you like.

TIP

Dissipate a glut: Carrot & roast pepper purée

In a pan with the lid on, gently prepare dinner 300g sliced carrots in a touch butter and 1 tablespoon water for 30 minutes until softened. Grill 1 halved purple pepper until charred. Go away in a plastic bag for 10 minutes, then peel off the skin and do away with the seeds. Whizz the carrots and pepper with 1 tablespoon purple wine vinegar until easy. Serve the purée with hen or lamb chops.

Quick Gazpacho

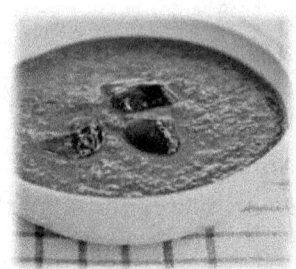

Full of vitamin C, low fat and counts as of your 5 a day – this must be at the menu every week!

- Cook: 10 minutes
- Serves: 1 servings

INGREDIENTS
- 250g passata
- 1 red pepper, deseeded and chopped
- 1 red chili, deseeded and chopped
- 1 garlic clove, crushed
- 1 teaspoon sherry vinegar
- juice ½ lime

DIRECTIONS

In a blender (or with a stick blender), whizz collectively the passata, purple pepper, chili, garlic, sherry vinegar and lime juice till soft. Season to flavor, and then serve with ice cubes.

Rich Tomato Soup With Pesto

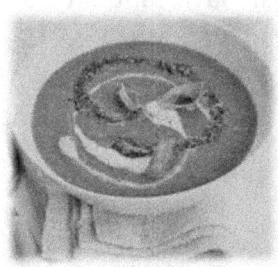

While you've got wealthy tinned tomatoes and intense, fruity Sun Blush tomatoes, there's no motive no longer to experience self-made tomato soup within the depths of wintry weather.

- Preparation: 10 minutes
- Cook: 15 minutes
- Serves: 4 servings

INGREDIENTS

☐ 1 tablespoon butter or olive oil
☐ 2 garlic cloves, crushed
☐ 5 soft sun-dried or Sun Blush tomatoes in oil, roughly chopped
☐ 3 x 400g cans plum tomatoes
☐ 500ml turkey or vegetable stock
☐ 1 teaspoon sugar, any type, or extra to taste
☐ 142ml pot soured cream
☐ 125g pot fresh basil pesto
☐ basil leaves, to serve

DIRECTIONS

1. Preheat the butter or oil in a big pan, then upload the garlic and melt for a few minutes over low warmth. Upload the sun-dried or Sun Blush tomatoes, canned tomatoes, inventory, sugar and seasoning, then deliver to a simmer. Let

the soup bubble for 10 minutes till the tomatoes have broken down a bit.

2. Whizz with a stick blender, adding half the pot of soured cream as you cross. Flavor and alter the seasoning – upload extra sugar in case you want to. Serve in bowls with 1 tablespoon or so of the pesto swirled on top, a touch greater soured cream and scatter with basil leaves.

TIP

Provide it a twist

Hearty rice & Seafood soup warmness 2 tablespoons oil from the sun-dried/Sun Blush tomatoes in a big saucepan. Add 185g sliced chorizo and 1 sliced onion and fry till golden. Observe the recipe above, leaving out the soured cream and pesto, then upload the chorizo and onion, alongside 85g paella rice. Simmer for 20mins till the rice is gentle (upload a bit water if it gets too thick), tip in a defrosted 400g bag mixed seafood. as soon as hot, serve in bowls scattered with chopped parsley.

Spicy Pasta Soup

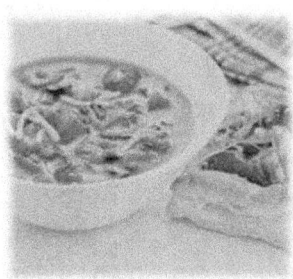

Rustle up an Italian-style minestrone soup and individual cakes using substances out of your store cupboard

- Preparation: 10 minutes
- Cook: 35 minutes
- Serves: 4 servings

INGREDIENTS
- ☐ 1 tablespoon olive oil, plus more for drizzling
- ☐ 1 red onion, finely chopped
- ☐ 1 red chili, deseeded and finely sliced
- ☐ 800g can whole plum tomatoes
- ☐ 1l vegetable stock
- ☐ 100g broken spaghetti
- ☐ 4 tablespoons chopped pitted black olives
- ☐ 2 tablespoons chopped capers, drained and rinsed
- ☐ large handful basil leaves, roughly torn, or 1 tablespoons pesto

DIRECTIONS
1. Preheat the oil in a big heavy-based totally saucepan. Upload the onion and chili, then cook dinner for 10 minutes till softened. Stir inside the tomatoes, breaking up with a spoon as you cross, and then pour within the stock. Cowl, carry to the boil, cast off the lid, then simmer for 5 minutes.

2. Upload the spaghetti, and then simmer for 6-8 minutes till it is just cooked. Stir in the olives, capers and basil or pesto, then serve drizzled with olive oil.

TIP

Antipasto brownies

Warmness oven to 190C/fan 170C/gasoline 5. Divide a 375g % equipped-rolled puff pastry into eight rectangles. Switch to a baking sheet, then rating a 1cm border round the edges. Brush edges with a touch crushed egg, then bake for 15 minutes till risen and golden. Lightly squash the risen Centre's. Spread with 3 tablespoons sparkling pesto, then pinnacle with 200g blended antipasto (inclusive of pink peppers and artichokes; we used Scala). Scatter on basil and rocket leaves, and then serve.

Hearty Mushroom Soup

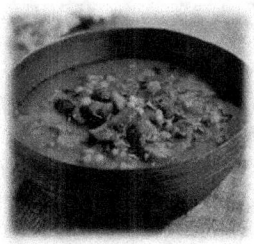

A fulfilling and low-fat vegetarian soup it really is a very good supply of folic acid

- Preparation: 30 minutes
- Cook: 30 minutes
- Serves: 6 servings

INGREDIENTS

☐ 25g pack porcini mushrooms
☐ 2 tablespoons olive oil
☐ 1 medium onion, finely diced
☐ 2 large carrots, diced
☐ 2 garlic cloves, finely chopped
☐ 1 tablespoon chopped rosemary, or 1 tsp dried
☐ 500g fresh mushrooms, for example chestnut, finely chopped
☐ 1.2l vegetable stock (from a cube is fine)
☐ 5 tablespoons marsala or dry sherry
☐ 2 tablespoons tomato purée
☐ 100g pearl barley
☐ grated fresh parmesan, to serve (elective)

DIRECTIONS

1. Positioned the porcini in a bowl with 250ml boiling water and depart to soak for 25 minutes. Warmth the oil in a pan and upload the onion, carrot, garlic, rosemary and seasoning.

Fry for 5 minutes on a medium heat till softened. Drain the porcini, saving the liquid, and finely chop. Tip into the pan with the fresh mushrooms. Fry for some other five minutes, then add the stock, Marsala or sherry, tomato purée, barley and strained porcini liquid.

2. Prepared for 30 minutes or till barley is tender, including more liquid if it becomes too thick. Serve in bowls with parmesan sprinkled over, if wanted.

Part 2

Quick Chilled Pea Soup

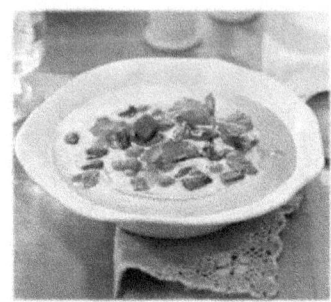

Blending a handful of spinach into the soup enhances the green color and adds subtle earthy notes.

PREP TIME: 18 mins

TOTAL TIME: 18 mins

YIELD: 4 servings

Quick Chilled Pea Soup

Ingredients
1 (14.4-ounce) package frozen petite green peas
¼ cup of water
2 cups of fresh baby spinach
1 ½ teaspoons of extra-virgin olive oil
1 minced garlic clove
1 teaspoon of extra-virgin olive oil,
1 cup of iced water
1 teaspoon of chopped fresh mint
1 tablespoon of fresh lemon juice
¼ teaspoons of salt
2 tablespoons of half-and-half
¼ teaspoon of freshly grinded black pepper

Preparation
1. Reserve ½ cup of peas from package.

2. Place remaining peas and ¼ cup water in a microwave-safe dish.
3. Cover with plastic wrap and pierce once with a knife to vent.
4. Microwave at high heat setting 5 minutes and add the spinach
5. Cover and microwave at high heat setting 2 minutes.
6. Drain and rinse well with cold water.
7. While the pea is boiling: heat a small skillet over medium-high heat setting.
8. Add 1 ½ teaspoons of extra-virgin olive oil to pan then swirl to coat.
9. Add the reserved ½ cup of peas and 1 minced garlic clove then cook for 4 minutes or until peas begin to brown and stir it frequently.
10. Add the spinach mixture, 1 tablespoon of extra-virgin olive oil, 1 minced garlic clove, 1 cup ice water, chopped fresh mint, fresh lemon juice, and salt into a blender and blend until smooth for about 4 minutes.
11. Add the half-and-half and blend until it is all mixed.
12. Pour about ¾ cup of soup into each of 4 bowls and sprinkle evenly with cooked peas and freshly grinded black pepper.

Black Bean Soup

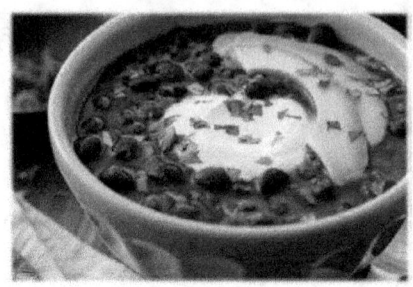

Black Bean Soup provides a hearty one-pot meal by itself, but we also like to serve this soup with tortillas or cheese tortillas.

SOAK TIME: 4 hours

PREP TIME: 10 mins

TOTAL TIME: 1 hour 45 mins

YIELD: 4 servings

Black Bean Soup

Ingredients
1 cup of dried black beans
2 teaspoons of vegetable oil
½ chopped medium onion,
1 teaspoon of chili powder
1 teaspoon of cumin, optional
1 14.5-oz. can of diced tomatoes with chilies
1 teaspoon of salt
1 teaspoon of lime or lemon juice, optional
low heat setting-fat sour cream, salsa and cilantro for garnish

Preparation

1. Rinse the beans under running water and pick through, while discarding any stones.

2. Place beans in a large pan and cover with 3 cups of water and allow it to boil.
3. Boil for 2 to 3 minutes and Reduce the Heat then cover and wait for 4 hours.
4. Rinse the beans and drain it.
5. Place beans in a large, clean pot, and pour fresh cold water over until it is covered by 1 inch then allow it to boil.
6. Reduce the heat and cook until beans are soft, about 1 ½ hours.
7. Let it cool off for 30 minutes.
8. Warm the oil in large pan over medium heat setting.
9. Cook the onion and stir it, until it begins to soften, for 2 to 3 minutes.
10. Add the chili powder and cumin, if desired and cook for 1 minute.
11. Add tomatoes, beans, salt and 1 cup water then boil.
12. Reduce the heat to medium low heat setting, and cover it.
13. Cook for 10 minutes and Reduce the Heat.
14. Add 1 Tbsp. of juice, if desired.
15. Top with low heat setting-fat sour cream, salsa or chopped cilantro before serving, if desired.

Caramelized Onion And Shiitake Soup With Gruyère–Blue Cheese Toasts

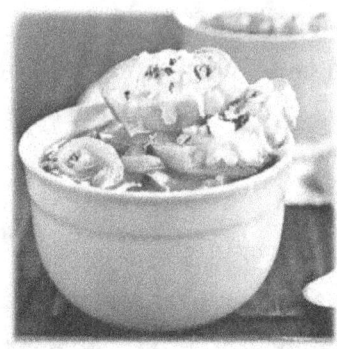

Earthy shiitake mushrooms and pungent cheese toasts give this soup more heartiness than classic French onion soup. For a light main course option, pair with a salad that's lightly dressed so it doesn't overpower the soup.

YIELD: 6 servings

Caramelized Onion and Shiitake Soup with Gruyère–Blue Cheese Toasts

Ingredients

Soup:
1 teaspoon of olive oil
cups of vertically sliced yellow onion (about 2 pounds)
cups of sliced shiitake mushroom caps (about 10 ounces' whole mushrooms)
minced garlic cloves
2 thyme sprigs
½ cup of dry white wine
1 (14-ounce) can of fat-free, less-sodium chicken broth
1 (14-ounce) can of fat-free, less-sodium beef broth
½ teaspoons of salt
½ teaspoon of freshly grinded black pepper

Toasts:

(½ -inch-thick) slices French bread baguette, toasted (about 6 ounces)
¼ cup (1 ounce) of grated Gruyère cheese
¼ cup (1 ounce) of crumbled Gorgonzola
½ teaspoon of finely of chopped fresh thyme
Preparation

To prepare soup:

1. Heat the oil in a large Dutch oven over medium-high heat setting.
2. Add onion to the oil in the pan and cook for 15 minutes or until almost soft and stir it frequently.
3. Reduce the heat to medium low heat setting and cook until it turns deep golden brown for about 40 minutes, and stir occasionally.
4. Increase heat to medium and add mushrooms to pan then cook for 10 minutes or until mushrooms are soft and stir it frequently.
5. Add garlic and thyme sprigs and cook for 2 minutes, and stir frequently.
6. Increase heat to medium-HIGH heat setting and add the wine to the pan then cook for 2 minutes or until most of the liquid evaporates.
7. Add the broths and allow it to boil then reduce the heat and cook for 45 minutes.
8. Add salt and pepper and discard thyme sprigs.

To prepare toasts:

1. Preheat broiler.
2. Arrange the bread in a single layer on a baking sheet.

3. Top each bread slices with 1 teaspoon of Gruyère and 1 teaspoon of Gorgonzola.
4. Broil for 2 minutes or until the cheese melts.
5. Sprinkle the chopped thyme over cheese.
6. Serve about 1 cup of soup into each of 6 bowls and top each serving with 2 toasts.

Lemon, Orzo, And Meatball Soup

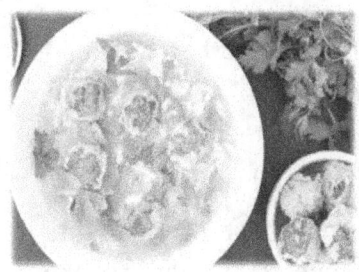

Lemon, Orzo, and Meatball Soup is our hearty twist on chicken noodle soup, featuring small grains of orzo pasta and savory chicken meatballs.

YIELD: Make about 6 quarts

Lemon, Orzo, and Meatball Soup

Ingredients
1-pound of grinded chicken
1 lightly beaten large egg
¼ cup of fine, dry breadcrumbs
1 teaspoon of kosher salt
teaspoons of loosely divided packed lemon zest
1 teaspoon of divided dried crushed rosemary
tablespoons of divided olive oil
1 medium-size of chopped sweet onion
thinly sliced carrots
2 minced garlic cloves
2 (32-oz.) containers of chicken broth
to 6 Tbsp. of lemon juice
¾ cup of orzo pasta
¼ cup of freshly grated Parmesan cheese
½ cup of fresh flat-leaf parsley leaves
Preparation

1. Add first 4 ingredients, 2 tsp. of lemon zest, and ½ tsp. rosemary in a medium bowl.
2. Shape into 30 (1-inch) meatballs (about 1 level tablespoonful of each).
3. Cook the meatballs, in 2 batches, in 1 Tbsp. of hot oil per batch in a Dutch oven over medium heat setting 3 to 4 minutes or until browned.
4. Remove using a slotted spoon.
5. Cook the onion and next 2 ingredients in remaining 1 Tbsp. hot oil in Dutch oven over medium-high heat setting for 3 to 5 minutes or until soft.
6. Add the broth, lemon juice, and remaining 2 tsp. of zest and ½ tsp. of rosemary and then allow it to boil and stir it occasionally.
7. Add the orzo then reduce heat to medium and cook and stir it occasionally, for 7 to 9 minutes or until pasta is almost soft.
8. Add the meatballs and cook for 5 to 7 minutes or until meatballs are thoroughly cooked.
9. Add salt and pepper to make it tasty.
10. Top with cheese and parsley.

Posole (Tomatillo, Chicken, And Hominy Soup)

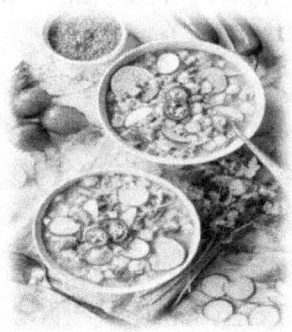

This Mexican soup was rated 5 stars because it's quick and packed with flavor. One reader called this Posole recipe "a Mexican chicken noodle soup."

YIELD: 8 servings (serving size: 1 ½ cups of soup, 1 teaspoon of cilantro, 1 ½ of teaspoons of sour cream, and 1 lime wedge)

Posole (Tomatillo, Chicken, and Hominy Soup)

Ingredients
1 pound of tomatillos
Cups of Brown Chicken Stock
2 cups of chopped onion
pounds of skinned chicken breast halves
chopped garlic cloves
2 seeded and quartered jalapeño peppers,
1 (30-ounce) can of drained white hominy
1 teaspoon of salt
½ cup of chopped fresh cilantro
¼ cup of reduced-fat sour cream
lime wedges

Preparation

1. Discard the husks and stems from the tomatillos.
2. Cook whole tomatillos in boiling water for 10 minutes or until soft then drain.
3. Place the tomatillos in a blender and it is process until smooth the set it aside.
4. Place the stock and the next 5 ingredients (stock through hominy) in a large stockpot then allow it to boil.
5. Cover and reduce the heat, and let it for cook 35 minutes or until chicken is done.
6. Remove chicken from its bones and shred.
7. Add the blended tomatillos and salt and cook for 5 minutes or until heated.
8. Add the chicken, and serve with cilantro, sour cream, and lime wedges.

Hot And Sour Shrimp Soup

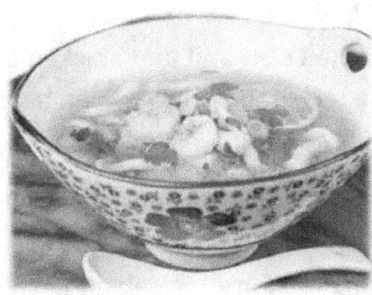

With its lively dance of flavors, this soup is a spring tonic.

TOTAL TIME: 30 mins

YIELD: 4 servings

Hot and Sour Shrimp Soup

Ingredients
2 lemongrass stalks
6 cups of reduced-sodium chicken broth
1 or 2 halved lengthwise serrano chilies
1 sliced shallot
2 slices (¼ in. thick) of crushed fresh ginger
1 small zucchini, cut into ½ -in. dice
4 button of quartered mushrooms
1 thinly sliced red jalapeño chili
¾ pound (about 50 per lb.) of small peeled and deveined raw shrimp,
1 teaspoon of Vietnamese or Thai fish sauce
About 1 tbsp. of white vinegar
¼ cup of cilantro leaves
2 tablespoons of coarsely chopped fresh dill
Preparation

1. Trim the green tips from the lemongrass and peel off tough outer layer from each.
2. Mash the stalks with a meat mallet or rolling pin, then tie each stalk in a knot.
3. Put them in a small pot, and add chicken broth, serrano chili, shallot, and ginger, then boil over high heat Setting.
4. Reduce the heat to medium and cook for 10 minutes.
5. Remove the lemongrass, serrano chili, and ginger from the pot then discard.
6. Add the zucchini, mushrooms, jalapeño chili, and shrimp.
7. Turn off the heat and make it steep until the shrimp is cooked through, for 2 minutes.
8. At the fish sauce, 1 tbsp. of vinegar, the cilantro, and dill.
9. Add more vinegar to make it tasty, if you like.
10. Divide among 4 bowls and serve hot.

Black Bean Soup With Chorizo And Lime

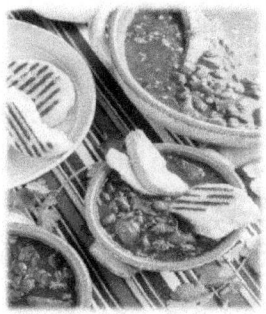

Smoky chorizo and bright lime add depth to a soup made quick with Canned beans.

YIELD: 4 servings

Black Bean Soup with Chorizo and Lime

Ingredients
2 teaspoons of divided olive oil
3 ounces of Spanish chorizo, quartered lengthwise and cut into ½ -inch pieces
1 cup of chopped onion
1 cup of chopped red bell pepper
2 teaspoons of chopped fresh oregano
2 teaspoons of minced garlic
1 teaspoon of grinded cumin
½ teaspoon of chipotle chili powder
¼ teaspoons of salt
2 cups of unsalted chicken stock (such as Swanson)
2 (15-ounce) CANs of rinsed, drained, and coarsely mashed unsalted black beans,
1 teaspoon of fresh lime juice
¼ cup of reduced-fat sour cream

¼ cup of chopped fresh cilantro

Preparation

1. Heat a large saucepan over medium heat setting.
2. Add 1 teaspoon of oil to pan and swirl to coat.
3. Add the chorizo and cook for 3 minutes and stir it occasionally.
4. Remove the chorizo from the pan (do not wipe pan).
5. Add the remaining 1 teaspoon of oil to the pan and swirl to coat.
6. Add onion and bell pepper and cook 3 minutes and stir it occasionally.
7. Add the oregano and the next 4 ingredients (through salt) and cook for 30 seconds.
8. Add the stock and beans, then boil, reduce the heat, and cook for 3 minutes.
9. Add the cooked chorizo and the juice.
10. Serve 1 ¼ cups of soup into each of 4 bowls and top each serving with 1 teaspoon of sour cream and 1 teaspoon of cilantro.

Cauliflower Soup With Shiitakes

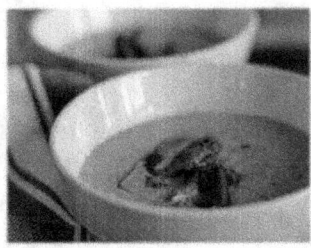

Smoky chorizo and bright lime add depth to a soup made quick with Canned beans.

HANDS-ON TIME: 35 mins

TOTAL TIME: 35 mins

YIELD: 4 servings

Cauliflower Soup with Shiitakes

Ingredients
4 teaspoons of divided extra-virgin olive oil
¾ cup of thinly sliced white and light green parts only leek
3/8 teaspoon of kosher salt, divided
4 cups of coarsely chopped Cauliflower florets (about 1 medium head)
1 ½ cups of unsalted chicken stock (such as Swanson), divided
¾ cup of water
2 teaspoons of chopped fresh thyme
¼ cup of 2% reduced-fat milk
1 ½ teaspoons of butter
¼ teaspoon of white pepper
1 (3.5-ounce) package of shiitake mushroom caps
1 teaspoon of low heater-sodium Worcestershire sauce
1 teaspoon ofherry vinegar
2 teaspoons of chopped fresh parsley

Preparation

1. Heat a large saucepan over high heat Setting.
2. Add 2 teaspoons of oil to pan and swirl to coat.
3. Add the leek and cook for 1 minute.
4. Add 1/8 teaspoons of salt.
5. Cover and reduce the heat to low heat setting, and cook for 5 minutes or until leeks are softened and stir it occasionally.
6. Add the Cauliflower 1 cup and 6 tablespoons of stock, ¾ cup of water, and thyme.
7. Then allow it to boil, cover and reduce heat, then for cook 7 minutes or until Cauliflower is very soft.
8. Place the Cauliflower mixture in a blender.
9. Remove center piece of blender lid (to allow steam to escape) secure blender lid and place a clean towel over opening in blender lid (to avoid splatters).
10. Blend the Cauliflower mixture until it is smooth.
11. Return the Cauliflower mixture to the saucepan.
12. Add remaining ¼ teaspoons of salt, milk, butter, and pepper.
13. And Keep it warm.
14. Thinly slice mushroom caps, heat a large skillet over medium-high heat setting.
15. Add remaining 2 teaspoons of oil to pan, and swirl to coat.
16. Add mushrooms and cook 6 minutes or until browned.
17. Add remaining 2 tablespoons of stock, Worcestershire sauce, and sherry vinegar and cook for 1 minute or until liquid is reduced and syrupy.
18. Spoon about 1 cup of soup into each of 4 bowls.
19. Top each serving with about 2 tablespoons of the mushroom mixture and sprinkle evenly with parsley.

Broccoli-Cheddar Soup

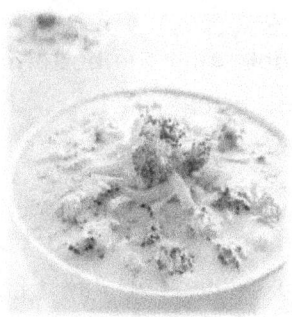

Hearty and satisfying, this soup gets its rich creaminess from potatoes.

TOTAL TIME: 38mins

YIELD: Serves 6 (serving size: 1 cup soup)

Broccoli-Cheddar Soup

Ingredients
4 cups of cubed peeled baking potato
½ teaspoon of divided salt
3 tablespoons of unsalted butter
1 cup of chopped onion
1/3 cup of chopped carrot
1 minced garlic clove,
5 cups of chopped divided fresh broccoli florets
3 cups of fat-free, low heater-sodium chicken broth
2 cups of plus 2 tablespoons of water, divided
2 cups of 1% low heat setting-fat milk
4 ounces of shredded reduced-fat sharp cheddar cheese, (about 1 cup)
Preparation

1. Place the potato and ¼ teaspoons of salt in a large saucepan and cover with water and allow it to boil.
2. Reduce the heat, and cook for 10 minutes or until soft then drain it.
3. While potatoes cook, melt the butter in a large Dutch oven over medium heat setting.
4. Cook the onion, carrot, and garlic for 5 minutes or until soft.
5. Add 4 cups of broccoli, broth, 2 cups of water, and ¼ teaspoons of salt and allow it to boil, and cook for 10 minutes or until broccoli is soft.
6. Add the potatoes, 1 cup of broccoli and 2 tablespoons of water in a microwave-safe bowl.
7. Cover it with plastic wrap and vent.
8. Microwave at high heat setting for 1 minute or until it turns bright green and make it drain.
9. Process the mixture in the Dutch oven with a hand-held immersion blender until smooth or place half of the broccoli mixture in a blender.
10. Remove the center piece of blender lid (to allow steam to escape) secure blender lid the place a clean towel over opening in blender lid (to avoid splatters).
11. Blend until smooth and pour it into a large bowl.
12. Repeat the procedure with the remaining broccoli mixture and return the mixture to Dutch oven.
13. Add milk and cheese and cook over low heat setting for 2 minutes and stir it until cheese melts and soup is smooth.
14. Add steamed broccoli.
15. Serve soup into individual bowls.

Two-Mushroom Velouté

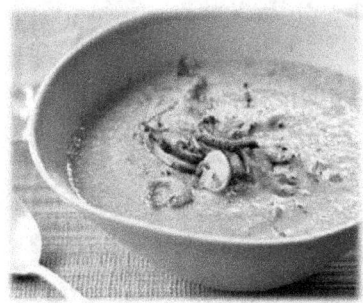

The secret to this mushroom soup: a little crème fraîche.

TOTAL TIME: 40 mins

YIELD: Serves 6

Two-Mushroom Velouté

Ingredients
1 ¼ pounds of white mushrooms
1 pound of finely chopped white mushrooms
¼ pound thinly sliced white mushrooms
1 teaspoon of fresh lemon juice
4 ½ cups of chicken stock or low heat setting-sodium broth
1-pound of stems discarded and caps and finely chopped shiitake mushrooms
2 minced large garlic cloves
2 teaspoons of vegetable oil
Salt and freshly grinded pepper
¼ cup of crème fraîche
1 ½ teaspoons of grinded coriander
Chopped chervil or parsley, for garnish

Preparation

1. Toss the chopped white mushrooms with the lemon juice in a bowl.

2. Add the chicken stock with the chopped white and shiitake mushrooms and the garlic and then boil them in a large saucepan.
3. Cook over Moderately low heat setting until it is the mushrooms are soft, for about 10 minutes.
4. Meanwhile, heat the oil in a medium nonstick skillet and add the sliced white mushrooms then cook over Moderately high heat Setting and stir it, until it turns golden brown and soft, for about 4 minutes.
5. Season it with salt and pepper.
6. Working in batches, blend the soup in a blender and blend until it turns very smooth
7. Return to the saucepan and mix in the crème fraîche.
8. Cook for 2 minutes and add the coriander and season it with salt and pepper.
9. Serve the soup into bowls.
10. Garnish with the cooked mushrooms and chervil then serve.

Pozole

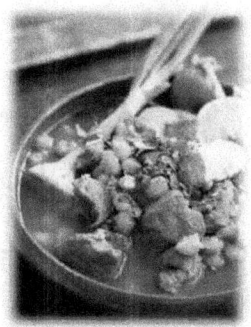

Serve the fresh garnishes with Bill Smith's earthy soup to add color and crunch.

PREP TIME: 1 hour

TOTAL TIME: 4 hours 5 mins

YIELD: 6 to 8 servings

Pozole

Ingredients
6 qt. of water
1 (3-lb.) whole chicken
1 pound of tomatillos with husks removed
2 stemmed jalapeño peppers
1 chopped medium-size yellow onion
6 garlic cloves
1 (28-oz.) CAN of crushed tomatoes
1 (29-oz.) CAN of drained Mexican-style or other Canned hominy,
2 tablespoons of dried Mexican oregano
4 dried bay leaves
2 dried stemmed cascabel chilies,
½ cup of hot water
2 teaspoons of salt

Lime wedges

Garnishes:
Fresh cilantro, sliced radishes, shredded cabbage

Preparation
1. Boil 6 qt. of water over high heat Setting in an 8-qt. stockpot.
2. Remove neck and giblets from chicken.
3. Add chicken, neck, and giblets to the boiling water and cook for 15 minutes.
4. Reduce the Heat, and wait for 20 minutes.
5. Transfer chicken to a plate, reserving the broth in stockpot then discard neck and giblets.
6. Cover and wait till the chicken cools down for about 30 minutes.
7. Meanwhile, Add the tomatillos, the next 3 ingredients, and 2 ½ cups of reserved broth in a medium saucepan.
8. Boil over medium-HIGH heat setting, and cook, will and stir occasionally, for 20 minutes or until garlic is very soft.
9. Separate the Skin and the bone of the chicken and reserve and any available juices.
10. Add the skin, bones, and juices to broth in stockpot and boil over medium-high heat setting and cook for about 30 to 45 minutes or until the bones begin to separate.
11. Pour mixture through a fine wire-mesh strainer into a large bowl, discarding solids particles then Return it to the pot.
12. Skim the fat from the broth and make broth cook over medium-HIGH heat setting.
13. Process the tomatillo mixture in a blender or food processor until smooth.
14. Add crushed tomatoes and the next 3 ingredients and stir it until it blends then allow it to boil.

15. Reduce the heat to medium low heat setting then cover it then cook and stir it occasionally for 1 hour.
16. Meanwhile, soak the chilies in ½ cup of hot water in a small bowl for 30 minutes.
17. Drain and reserve the soaking liquid.
18. Process chilies and 2 to 3 Tbsp. of soaking liquid in a blender or food processor until it turns smooth.
19. Add 2 tsp. salt and pepper to make it tasty into broth.
20. Pour chili mixture through a fine wire-mesh strainer into broth, while discarding the solid particles.
21. Add the shredded chicken, and cook for 15 minutes.
22. When done, Serve with lime wedges.

Red Lentil-Pumpkin Soup

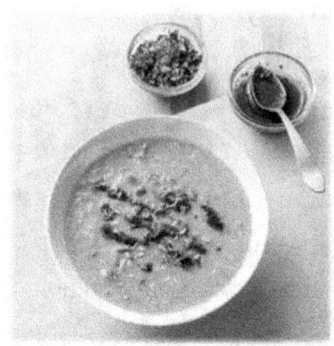

The hearty crunch of pumpkin seed adds wonderful contrast to this rich, creamy soup.

PREP TIME: 28 mins

TOTAL TIME: 28 mins

YIELD: 4 servings

Red Lentil-Pumpkin Soup

   Ingredients
2 teaspoons of Canola oil
1 cup of chopped onion
1 teaspoon of minced garlic
3 ½ cups of divided organic vegetable broth
1 cup of dried small red lentils
1 teaspoon of grinded cumin
¼ teaspoons of salt
¼ teaspoon of grinded cinnamon
1/8 teaspoon of grinded red pepper
1 cup of water
¾ cup of Canned pumpkin
1 teaspoon of grated peeled fresh ginger
1 teaspoon of fresh lemon juice

3 tablespoons of plain low heat setting-fat yogurt
¼ cup of unsalted pumpkinseed kernels, toasted
¼ cup of chopped fresh cilantro

Preparation

1. Heat a large Dutch oven over medium-high heat setting.
2. Add oil to the pan and swirl to coat.
3. Add onion and garlic to the pan and cook 4 minutes.
4. Add 3 cups of broth, lentils, and the next 4 ingredients (through red pepper) then boil.
5. Reduce heat, and cook for 10 minutes or until lentils are soft.
6. Place the lentil mixture in a blender and remove the center piece of blender lid to allow steam to escape and secure the blender lid, then place a clean towel over opening in blender lid to avoid splatters. Blend until it turns smooth.
7. Return the lentil mixture to the pan over medium heat setting.
8. Add the remaining ½ cup of broth, 1 cup of water, and pumpkin to the pan then cook 3 minutes or until thoroughly heated.
9. Add the ginger and lemon juice.
10. Serve 1 ½ cups of soup into each of 4 bowls and top each serving with about 2 teaspoons of yogurt, 1 tablespoon of pumpkinseeds, and 1 tablespoon of cilantro.

Thai Chicken Soup

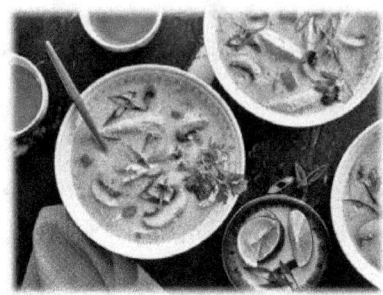

For a quick dinner that's full of distinctive Thai flavor, offer Thai Chicken Soup.

TOTAL TIME: 40 mins

YIELD: 4 servings

Thai Chicken Soup

Ingredients
1 teaspoon of olive oil
3 tablespoons of minced shallots
2 tablespoons of minced fresh garlic
1 teaspoon of grated peeled fresh ginger
1 (14.5-ounce) can of fat-free, low heater-sodium chicken broth
3 (5-inch) pieces of peeled fresh lemongrass, crushed
2 cups of water
2 cups of shredded skinless, boneless rotisserie chicken breast
2 cups of chopped bok choy
¼ cup of fresh cilantro leaves
¼ cup of small fresh basil leaves
2 tablespoons of fresh lime juice
¼ teaspoons of salt
2 cups of hot cooked whole-grain rice noodles
1/8 teaspoon of crushed red pepper

Preparation

1. Heat a large saucepan over medium-high heat setting.
2. Add oil to the pan and swirl to coat.
3. Add the shallots and cook for 1 minute and stir it frequently.
4. Add garlic and ginger and cook for 30 seconds and stir it constantly.
5. Add the broth then boil, while scraping pan to loosen browned bits.
6. Add lemongrass and 2 cups of water to broth mixture then boil.
7. Reduce the heat and cook for 10 minutes.
8. Add the chicken and bok choy and cook for 5 minutes.
9. Discard lemongrass and Reduce the Heat
10. Add the cilantro, basil, lime juice, and salt.
11. Place ½ cup of noodles in each of 4 bowls and top each serving with 1 ¼ cups of soup.
12. Sprinkle with red pepper.

Beef Dumpling Soup

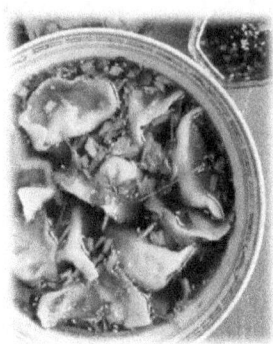

Are you looking for easy slow cooker soup recipes? Well, you've found what you need here. Beef Dumpling Soup is easy, delicious, and it's not your ordinary dumpling soup. It barely requires any preparation. If you use instant biscuit mix, the dumplings come together very quickly and are still extremely tasty. Plus, the combination of veggies and meat really complement each other and make this a balanced meal!

YIELD: 30 mins

SLOW COOKER TIME HIGH: 40 - 60 hours

SCLOW COOKER TIME LOW: 30 minutes

Beef Dumpling Soup

Ingredients

1-pound of cubed beef stew meat
1 package of Lipton's onion soup mix
6 cups of hot water
2 peeled and shredded carrots
1 stalk of finely chopped celery
1 peeled and chopped tomato
1 cup of biscuit mix
1 tablespoon of finely chopped parsley
6 tablespoons of milk

Preparation
1. 1-pound of cubed beef stew meat
2. 1 package of Lipton's onion soup mix
3. 6 cups of hot water
4. 2 peeled and shredded carrots
5. 1 stalk of finely chopped celery
6. 1 peeled and chopped tomato
7. 1 cup of biscuit mix
8. 1 tablespoon of finely chopped parsley
9. 6 tablespoons of milk
10. Instructions:
11. Add and sprinkle the beef with dry onion soup mix in a slow cooker.
12. Pour hot water over the meat and add the carrots, celery and tomato.
13. Cover and cook on low heat settings for 4-6 hours or until the meat is cooked.
14. Turn the control to high heat settings.
15. Combine the biscuit mix with parsley in a small bowl.
16. Add the milk with fork until the mixture is moistened.
17. Drop the dumpling mixture into slow cooker with a teaspoon.
18. Cover and cook on high heat settings for 30 minutes.

Spicy Coconut Shrimp Soup

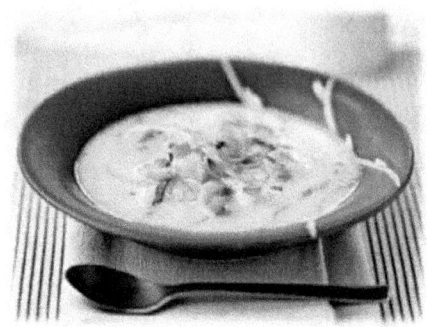

For a spicier finish to Spicy Coconut Shrimp Soup, top with minced Thai chili pepper.

PREP TIME: 55 mins

TOTAL TIME: 55 mins

YIELD: 4 to 6 servings

Spicy Coconut Shrimp Soup

Ingredients

1 pound of unpeeled, medium-size raw Gulf shrimp (36/40 count)
1 teaspoon of grated fresh ginger
4 minced garlic cloves
2 teaspoons of olive oil
4 cups of vegetable broth
1 (13.5-oz.) can of unsweetened coconut milk
2 ½ tablespoons of fish sauce
1 teaspoon of light brown sugar
1 teaspoon of fresh lime juice
2 teaspoons of red curry paste
1 (8-oz.) package of sliced fresh mushrooms
1 medium-size chopped red bell pepper

¼ cup of chopped fresh basil
¼ cup of chopped fresh cilantro
¼ cup of sliced green onions
1 seeded and minced Thai chili pepper(optional)

Preparation

1. Peel the shrimp
2. Cook the ginger and garlic in hot oil in a large Dutch oven over medium-high heat setting for 1 to 2 minutes or until fragrant.
3. Add the broth and the next 5 ingredients.
4. Boil the broth mixture and reduce heat to medium.
5. Add the mushrooms and bell pepper, and cook and stir it for 3 to 5 minutes or until crisp-soft.
6. Add the shrimp, and cook for 1 to 2 minutes or until shrimp turns pink.
7. Reduce the Heat and add basil, the next 2 ingredients, and, the chili pepper.

Roasted SQuash Soup With Sage

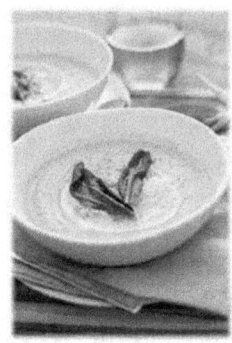

Roasted acorn squash and earthy sage sing in this delightful winter soup.

TOTAL TIME: 2 hours

YIELD: 8 servings

Roasted Squash Soup with Sage

Ingredients

8 medium of acorn squash (roundish)
4 tablespoons of mild extra-virgin olive oil
1 chopped medium yellow onion,
1 teaspoon of smoked paprika
2 tablespoons of chopped sage, plus several leaves for garnish
About 1 ½ tsp. of coarse sea salt
2 chopped garlic cloves,
5 to 6 cups of chicken broth
½ teaspoon of freshly grinded black pepper
½ cup of crème fraîche

Preparation

1. Preheat oven to 375°.
2. Cut the top third off each squash and scoop out the seeds from the squash bottoms and tops, then discard.

3. Trim the bottom of each squash so that it can sit straight.
4. Set the squash bottoms and tops on 2 large baking sheets and drizzle with about 2 tbsp. of oil, rubbing it all over the insides and rims.
5. Bake for 45 to 55 minutes, or until the flesh is soft and turns golden brown, but before squash start collapsing.
6. Meanwhile, heat the remaining 2 tbsp. of oil in a large pot over medium heat setting and add onion, paprika, sage, and ½ tsp. of salt then cook until it turns golden brown, for about 5 minutes.
7. Add garlic and cook for 2 minutes more.
8. Scoop the cooked flesh from squash into the pot, while leaving enough flesh so that the squash can maintain its shape.
9. Add 5 cups of stock, the remaining 1 tsp. of salt, and pepper and allow it to boil but reduce the heat and cook for 5 minutes.
10. Add salt to make it tasty.
11. Purée the soup in a blender, and add more stock if soup is too thick, cover top of the blender with a towel to keep hot soup from spurting out.
12. Reheat the soup in the pot and add the crème fraiche and more stock if necessary.
13. Serve soup into squash bowls and top with sage leaves.

Baby Carrot Soup

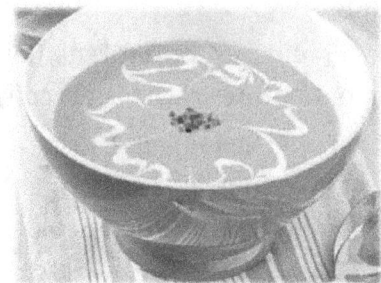

Smoky adobo sauce gives this creamy soup a subtle touch of heat.

PREP TIME: 10 mins

TOTAL TIME: 35 mins

YIELD: 5 cups of (serving size: 1 cup)

Baby Carrot Soup

Ingredients
1 (7-oz.) can of chipotle peppers in adobo sauce
1 small chopped sweet onion,
1 teaspoon of olive oil
1 (32-oz.) container of low heat setting-sodium fat-free chicken broth
1 (16-oz.) package of baby carrots
1/3 cup of half-and-half
1 teaspoon of salt

Toppings:
chopped fresh chives
chopped dried chili peppers
reduced-fat sour cream

Preparation

1. Remove 2 tsp. of the adobo sauce from the can and reserve the peppers and the remaining sauce for another use.
2. Cook the onion in hot oil in a Dutch oven over medium heat setting for 3 to 4 minutes or until it is soft.
3. Add the broth, carrots, and 2 tsp. of adobo sauce, cover it, and increase the heat to medium-high heat setting, and then start boiling.
4. Reduce the heat to medium, cover it partially and cook, for 15 to 20 minutes or until carrots are soft.
5. Reduce the Heat, and let it cool down for 10 minutes.
6. Process the carrot mixture in a blender or food processor for 1 minute or until it is smooth.
7. Return the carrot mixture to the Dutch oven.
8. Add the half-and-half and salt then cook over low heat setting for 2 to 4 minutes or until it is thoroughly heated.
9. Serve with desired toppings.

Cheeseburger Soup

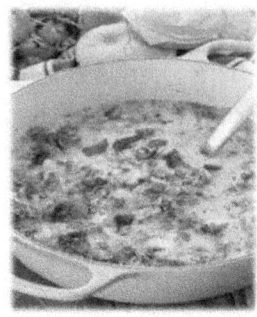

All the ingredients of your favorite cheeseburger are included in this chunky soup.
YIELD: 8 cups

Cheeseburger Soup

   Ingredients
2 cups of peeled and cubed potatoes
2 peeled and grated carrots
1 chopped onion
1 seeded and chopped jalapeno pepper
1 minced clove garlic
1 ½ cups of water
1 teaspoon of beef bouillon granules
½ teaspoons of salt
1-pound of browned and drained grinded beef
2 ½ cups of divided milk
3 tablespoons of all-purpose flour
1 8-oz. pkg. of cubed pasteurized process cheese spread,

Optional:
¼ to 1 teaspoon of cayenne pepper
Garnishes:

½ pound of crisply cooked and crumbled bacon

Preparation

1. Add the first 8 ingredients in a large saucepan then boil over medium heat setting.
2. Reduce the heat and cook until the potatoes are soft.
3. Add the grinded beef and 2 cups of milk.
4. Mix the flour and the remaining milk together in a small bowl until smooth it gradually mixes with soup.
5. Then boil and cook for 2 minutes or until thick and bubbly and stir it constantly.
6. Reduce the heat and add the cheese then stir until it melts.
7. Add the cayenne pepper, if desired.
8. Top it with bacon before serving.

Butternut SQuash-Parsnip Soup

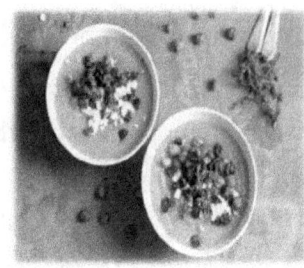

To serve 12, make two batches of soup instead of doubling the recipe.

PREP TIME: 15 mins

COOK TIME: 2 hrs 30 mins

STAND TIME: 1 hour

YIELD: 6 cups

Butternut Squash-Parsnip Soup

Ingredients
2 cups of peeled and cubed potatoes
2 peeled and grated carrots
1 chopped onion
1 seeded and chopped jalapeno pepper
1 minced clove garlic
1 ½ cups of water
1 teaspoon of beef bouillon granules
½ teaspoons of salt
1-pound of browned and drained grinded beef
2 ½ cups of divided milk
3 tablespoons of all-purpose flour
1 8-oz. pkg. of cubed pasteurized process cheese spread,

Optional:

¼ to 1 teaspoon of cayenne pepper

Garnishes:

½ pound of crisply cooked and crumbled bacon

Preparation

1. Melt the butter with olive oil in a large Dutch oven over medium heat setting and add the onion and the next 4 ingredients, then cook for 20 minutes or until the onion's color turns caramel.
2. Add the squash and chicken broth.
3. Then boil over medium-high heat setting, reduce heat to medium, and cook and stir it often for 10 minutes.
4. Remove the soup from heat and wait for 1 hour.
5. Process the squash mixture, in batches, by using a blender or food processor until it turns smooth.
6. Pour mixture into a 6-qt. slow cooker and add the whipping cream, paprika, and cumin.
7. Cover it and cook on low heat setting for 2 hours and stir it occasionally.
8. Garnish, if desired.
9. Preheat the oven to 400°.
10. Cut the squash in half and remove the seeds, cut the sides, on a lightly greased aluminum foil-lined baking sheet.
11. Bake it at 400° for 45 minutes or until squash pulp is soft.
12. Remove from oven and let it cool down for 20 minutes.
13. Scoop out squash pulp, and discard the shells.

Zucchini Soup

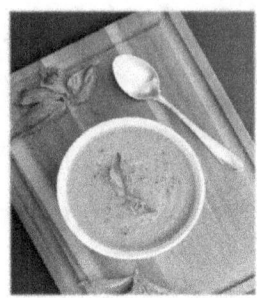

Your family won't notice the beans in this blended soup.

PREP TIME: 20 mins

COOK TIME: 25 mins

STAND TIME: 10 mins

YIELD: 7 cups of (serving size: 1 ½ cups)

Zucchini Soup

Ingredients
1 cup of chopped celery
1 cup of chopped onion
1 teaspoon of olive oil
1 ½ pounds of zucchini, cut into ¼ -inch pieces (about 5 cups)
3 cups of low heat setting-sodium chicken broth
1 (16-oz.) can of rinsed and drained Cannellini beans
1 teaspoon of salt
¼ teaspoons of seasoned pepper

Garnishes:
Thinly sliced radishes
crumbled feta cheese
Preparation

1. Cook the chopped celery and onion inside hot olive oil in a Dutch oven over medium-high heat setting 8 minutes or until it is soft.
2. Add the zucchini and the next 4 ingredients.
3. Then boil over medium heat setting and reduce heat to low heat setting, and cook for 10 minutes or until the zucchini is soft.
4. Remove it from heat, and wait for 20 minutes.
5. Process the soup, in batches, in a blender or food processor for 30 seconds or until it is smooth.
6. Return soup to the Dutch oven, and cook it over medium heat setting for 5 minutes or until it is thoroughly cooked.
7. Garnish, if desired.

Roasted Red Pepper Soup With Pesto Croutons

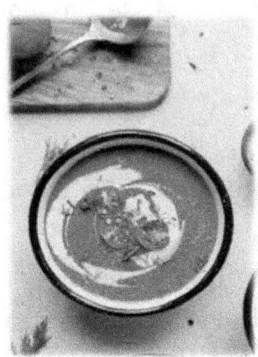

Your family won't notice the beans in this blended soup.

PREP TIME: 20 mins

COOK TIME: 35 mins

STAND TIME: 10 mins

YIELD: 6 servings

Roasted Red Pepper Soup with Pesto Croutons

Ingredients
¼ cup of refrigerated pesto, at room temperature
6 sourdough of bread slices
1 tablespoon of butter
1 tablespoon of olive oil
1 minced garlic clove
1 finely chopped shallot
1 tablespoon of tomato paste
1 (15-oz.) jar of rinsed and drained roasted red bell peppers
4 cups of LOW heat setting-sodium chicken broth
¼ cup of half-and-half
1 tablespoon of chopped fresh parsley
Salt and pepper to make it tasty

Garnishes:

Fresh flat-leaf parsley sprigs
Shaved parmesan cheese

Preparation

1. Preheat the oven at 350°.
2. Spread the pesto on 1 side of each bread slice.
3. Cut each bread slice into ½ - to 1-inch cubes.
4. Place bread cubes in a single layer on a lightly greased aluminum foil-lined jelly-roll pan.
5. Bake at 350° for 16 to 20 minutes or until it turns golden, turning it once after 10 minutes.
6. Remove from oven, and let it cool down.
7. Melt the butter with the oil in a large Dutch oven over medium-high heat setting.
8. Add the garlic and shallot, and cook and stir it constantly, for 2 minutes or until vegetables are soft.
9. Add the tomato paste, and cook and stir it constantly, for 1 minute.
10. Add the bell peppers and chicken broth, then boil.
11. Reduce the heat to medium, and cook and stir it occasionally, for 5 minutes.
12. Reduce the Heat let it cool down for 10 minutes.
13. Process the red pepper mixture, in batches, in a blender or food processor for 8 to 10 seconds until it turns smooth.
14. Return the red pepper mixture to the Dutch oven and add the half-and-half and parsley, and cook over medium heat setting for 5 minutes or until thoroughly heated.
15. Season it with salt and pepper to make it tasty.
16. Serve the soup into 6 bowls and top it with croutons.
17. Garnish, if desired.

Avocado Soup With Citrus-Shrimp Relish

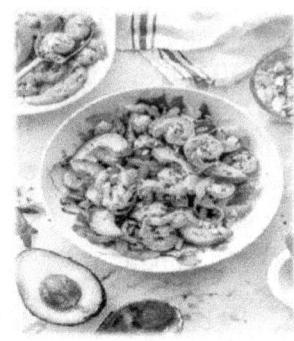

This lovely no-cook soup makes a refreshing entrée with a green salad.

YIELD: 4 servings

Avocado Soup with Citrus-Shrimp Relish

Ingredients

Relish:

2 tablespoons of chopped fresh cilantro
1 teaspoon of grated lemon rind
1 teaspoon of finely chopped red onion
1 teaspoon of extra virgin olive oil
8 ounces of peeled and deveined steamed and coarsely chopped medium shrimp

Soup:
2 cups of fat-free, less-sodium chicken broth
1 ¾ cups of chopped avocado (about 2)
1 cup of water
1 cup of rinsed and drained canned navy beans
½ cup of fat-free plain yogurt
1 ½ tablespoons of fresh lemon juice
¼ teaspoon of salt

¼ teaspoon of black pepper
¼ teaspoon of hot pepper sauce
1 small seeded and chopped jalapeño pepper
¼ cup (1 ounce) crumbled queso fresco cheese

Preparation

To prepare relish:

1. Add the first 5 ingredients in a small bowl, while tossing gently.

To prepare soup:

1. Add the broth and the next 9 ingredients (through jalapeño) in a blender and blend until it turns smooth.
2. Serve 1 ¼ cups of avocado the mixture into each of 4 bowls
3. Top each serving with ¼ cup shrimp mixture and 1 tablespoon of cheese.

Red Pepper-Cauliflower Soup

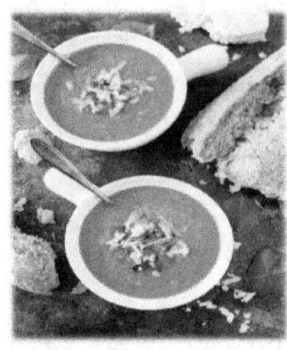

Red peppers give this Cauliflower soup gorgeous color and smooth texture.
TOTAL TIME: 1 hour

YIELD: 4 servings

Red Pepper-Cauliflower Soup

Ingredients
6 large stemmed and cored, halved lengthwise, and pressed flat red bell peppers
1 tablespoon of olive oil
4 peeled and chopped shallots
1 teaspoon of salt
¼ teaspoon of cayenne
1-quart fat-skimmed chicken broth
1 head Cauliflower, cut into florets
1 teaspoon of sugar
Freshly grinded pepper
Extra-virgin olive oil (optional)
Chopped fresh chives (optional)
Lemon wedges (optional)

Preparation

1. Preheat the broiler to high heat setting.

2. Arrange the bell peppers skin side up on baking sheet.
3. Broil, while watching carefully, until the skins are blackened, for about 10 minutes.
4. Remove the peppers from the oven and let it cool down.
5. Peel over a bowl in order to collect the juices then set the peppers and juices aside.
6. Warm the olive oil in a large pot over medium-high heat setting.
7. Add the shallots, salt, and cayenne and cook, and keep and stir until it gets soft, for 3 minutes.
8. Add the broth and Cauliflower then boil, and low heater heat.
9. Cover and cook for 20 minutes then add the peppers with the juices and cook until the Cauliflower is soft for 10 minutes.
10. Purée in batches in a blender then add sugar and add pepper to make it tasty.
11. Serve whether hot or cold
12. Garnish with a drizzle of extra-virgin olive oil, some chives, and a squeeze of lemon juice if you like.

Spicy Tomato And White Bean Soup

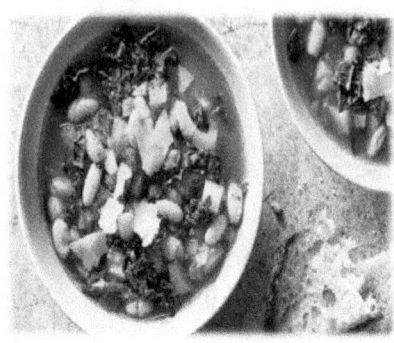

Pair this soup with a simple grilled cheese sandwich for a quick and satisfying meal.

YIELD: 4 servings (serving size: 1 cup)

Spicy Tomato and White Bean Soup

Ingredients
1 (14-ounce) of divided less-sodium fat-free chicken broth can
2 teaspoons of chili powder
1 teaspoon of grinded cumin
1 (16-ounce) CAN of drained and rinsed navy beans,
1 medium halved and seeded polao chili
½ onion, cut into ½-inch-thick wedges
1 pint of grape tomatoes
¼ cup of chopped fresh cilantro
2 tablespoons of fresh lime juice
1 tablespoon of extra virgin olive oil
½ teaspoon of salt
Cilantro sprigs (optional)

Preparation

1. Add 1 cup of broth, chili powder, cumin, and beans in a Dutch oven over medium-high heat setting.

2. Add the remaining broth, poblano, and onion in a food processor, and pulse until the vegetables are well chopped.
3. Add the onion mixture to the pan.
4. Add the tomatoes and cilantro to food processor, and process until it si coarsely chopped.
5. Add the tomato mixture to pan and boil.
6. Cover it, and reduce the heat, then cook for 5 minutes or until vegetables are soft.
7. Reduce the Heat and add the juice, olive oil, and salt.
8. Garnish with cilantro sprigs, if desired.

Green Onion Egg Drop Soup

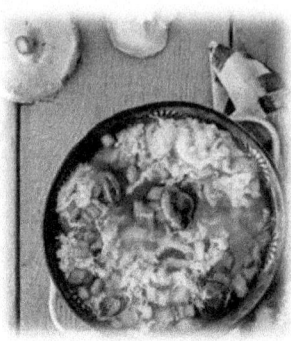

Egg drop soup is often garnished with a few sliced green onions, but this version uses a generous amount for a rich flavor. Mixed eggs are stirred into cooking broth to thicken the soup and create delicate ribbons.

YIELD: 4 cups of (serving size: 1 cup)

Green Onion Egg Drop Soup

Ingredients

3 cups of fat-free, less-sodium chicken broth
1 cup of water
½ cup of thinly sliced green onions
1/3 cup of thinly sliced shiitake mushroom caps
1 ½ teaspoons of low heat setting-sodium soy sauce
¼ teaspoon of grated peeled fresh ginger
2 large egg whites
1 large egg
Dash of freshly grinded black pepper

Preparation

1. Add the first 6 ingredients in a medium saucepan over medium-HIGH heat setting then boil.
2. Reduce the heat, and cook 3 minutes.

3. Add the egg whites and egg and stir with a mix.
4. Pour the egg mixture into cooking broth mixture and stir once.
5. Cook for 1 minute.
6. Reduce the Heat and add pepper.
7. Serve immediately.

Roasted Red Pepper Soup

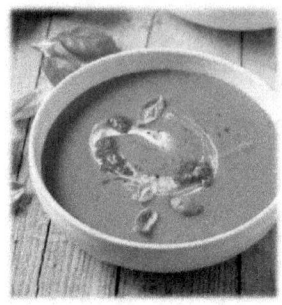

Jarred roasted red peppers give this comforting wintertime soup its rich flavor and color.

PREP TIME: 15 mins

COOK TIME: 30 mins

YIELD: 8 servings

Roasted Red Pepper Soup

Ingredients
1 stick (¼ lb.) of unsalted butter
6 finely chopped onions
4 minced cloves garlic
4 (14 oz.) cans of Italian plum tomatoes with their juice
(13.75 oz.) cans of chicken or vegetable broth
1 (15 oz.) can of crushed tomatoes
4 (7 oz.) jars of chopped roasted red peppers
2 tablespoons of Pernod or other anise-flavored liqueur (optional)
1 tablespoon of fresh thyme leaves, plus more for garnish
½ teaspoon of kosher salt
½ teaspoon of black pepper
1 cup of sour cream
2 teaspoons of grated lemon peel

Preparation

1. Melt butter over medium heat setting in a Dutch oven or other large, heavy pot.
2. Add the onions and cook and stir it, until it softens, for about 10 minutes.
3. Add the garlic and cook and stir it, for 2 minutes.
4. Add the plum tomatoes and their juice, chicken broth and crushed tomatoes then boil and cook for 5 minutes.
5. Add the red peppers, Pernod (if using), thyme, salt and pepper, then cook for 5 minutes additionally.
6. stir the sour cream and lemon peel together in a bowl, cover and refrigerate.
7. Strain the soup into a large bowl.
8. Blend strained solids in batches in a blender or food processor. Strain again over the same bowl and discard solids particles.
9. Wipe out Dutch oven, and add the soup and allow it to boil.
10. Strain the soup into a serving bowl, dollop sour cream on top and garnish with thyme.

Southwestern Chicken Soup

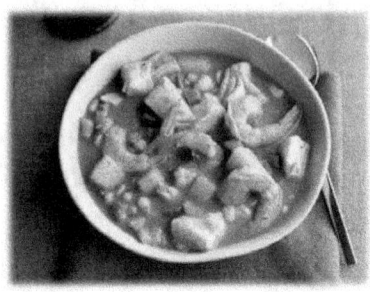

This top-rated Southwestern chicken soup is a great way to use up leftover chicken. The creamy chunks of avocado add a richness that's unusual to find in most chicken soups.

YIELD: 6 servings (serving size: 1 2/3 cups of soups and 1 lime wedge)

Southwestern Chicken Soup

Ingredients

Cooking spray
1 cup of chopped onion
3 minced garlic cloves
6 cups of fat-free, less-sodium chicken broth
¼ cup of uncooked white rice
1 teaspoon of grinded cumin
1 (16-ounce) can of rinsed and drained Great Northern beans
3 cups of chopped skinless, boneless rotisserie chicken breast
½ cup of coarsely chopped fresh cilantro
½ teaspoon of black pepper
¼ teaspoon of salt
1 cup chopped of seeded tomato
¾ cup of diced peeled avocado (about 1 medium)
1 tablespoon of fresh lime juice
6 lime wedges

Preparation

1. Heat a large cook pan over medium-high heat setting.
2. Coat pan with cooking spray.
3. Add onion and garlic, and cook for 3 minutes.
4. Add the broth, rice, cumin, and beans, then boil.
5. Reduce heat and cook 15 minutes.
6. Add the chicken, cilantro, pepper, and salt and cook for 5 minutes or until the chicken is thoroughly heated.
7. Reduce the Heat, and add the tomato, avocado, and juice.
8. Serve with lime wedges.

Thai Coconut Soup

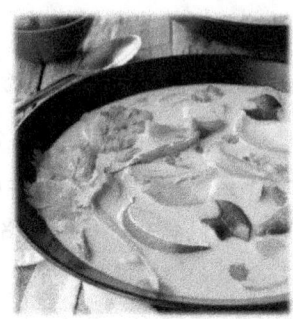

Seed the chilies if you prefer a milder soup.

PREP TIME: 10 mins

COOK TIME: 20 mins

YIELD: Make 7 cups

Thai Coconut Soup

Ingredients
4 cups of chicken broth
1 (15-ounce) CAN of coconut milk
1 tablespoon of fish sauce
1 (2-inch) piece of peeled and sliced fresh ginger
1 to 2 serrano or sliced jalapeño chilies
1 stalk lemon grass, cut into 1-inch pieces (optional)
2 to 3 kaffir lime leaves (optional)
2 tablespoons of fresh lime juice
½ pound of peeled and deveined shrimp or 1 (12-ounce) package of cubed extra-firm tofu
½ (8-ounce) package of sliced cremini or baby bella mushrooms
2 tablespoons of fresh cilantro leaves
Preparation

1. Add the first 5 ingredients and, if desired, lemon grass and kaffir lime leaves in a large saucepan over medium-HIGH heat setting.
2. Boil and reduce heat, and cook for 10 minutes.
3. Add lime juice and the shrimp, then cook for 10 more minutes.
4. Discard ginger and lemon grass.
5. Add sliced mushrooms and cilantro.

Tortilla Soup With Chorizo And Turkey Meatballs

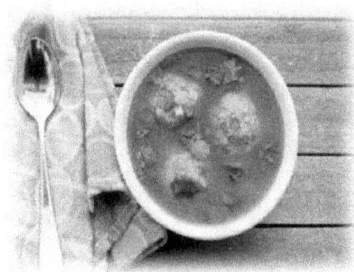

Smoked chorizo gives Tortilla Soup with Chorizo and Turkey Meatballs a deep, smoky flavor without overpowering. This Tortilla Soup is a perfect go-to for parties or quick get-togethers.
YIELD: Serves 4 (serving size: about 1 ½ cups)

Tortilla Soup with Chorizo and Turkey Meatballs

Ingredients
2 teaspoons of olive oil
1 cup of pre-chopped onion
¾ cup of chopped seeded poblano pepper
1 ounce of finely chopped smoked Spanish chorizo
4 cups of unsalted chicken stock
1 (14.5-ounce) CAN of unsalted drained diced tomatoes
2 chopped corn tortillas,
½ teaspoon of divided kosher salt
½ teaspoon of garlic powder
½ teaspoon of grinded cumin
½ teaspoon of grinded coriander
12 ounces 93% lean grinded turkey
1 large egg
Cooking spray

¾ cup frozen corn kernels
¼ cup chopped fresh cilantro

Preparation

1. Heat a large saucepan over medium-high heat setting.
2. Add the oil and swirl to coat.
3. Add the onion, poblano, and chorizo and for cook 2 minutes.
4. Add the stock and tomatoes and allow it to boil.
5. Add the tortillas and ¼ teaspoon of salt, garlic powder, and the next 4 ingredients (through egg).
6. Shape turkey mixture into 12 meatballs.
7. Heat a large skillet over medium-high heat setting.
8. Coat pan with cooking spray.
9. Add meatballs and cook for 4 minutes, while browning on all sides.
10. Add he meatballs, the remaining ¼ teaspoon of salt, and the corn to stock mixture, and cook for 5 minutes.
11. Serve and top with cilantro.

Curried Cauliflower Soup

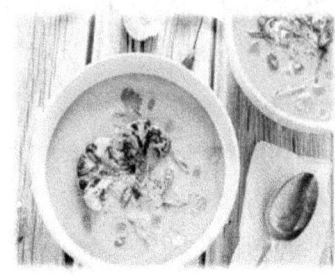

Smoked chorizo gives Tortilla Soup with Chorizo and Turkey Meatballs a deep, smoky flavor without overpowering. This Tortilla Soup is a perfect go-to for parties or quick get-togethers.
PREP TIME: 25 mins

TOTAL TIME: 1 hour 25 mins

YIELD: Serves 10 (serving size: 2/3 cup)

Curried Cauliflower Soup

Ingredients
1 ¾ pounds of Cauliflower (1 large head), cut into ½ -inch-thick slices
Cooking spray
¼ cup slivered almonds
1 ½ teaspoons of unsalted butter
¾ cup chopped yellow onion
3 crushed garlic cloves
1 peeled and chopped Granny Smith apple, (about 1 ½ cups)
1 ½ teaspoons of curry powder
4 cups of water
½ teaspoon of kosher salt
¼ teaspoon of black pepper
1 bay leaf
2/3 cup of half-and-half

¼ cup of plain 2% reduced-fat Greek yogurt
2 teaspoons of chopped fresh chives
Cracked black pepper

Preparation

1. Preheat oven to 375°.
2. Place the Cauliflower on a baking sheet coated with cooking spray.
3. Lightly coat the Cauliflower with cooking spray.
4. Bake at 375° for 30 minutes or until the Cauliflower begins to get brown on the bottom.
5. Turn the Cauliflower over and bake 5 minutes.
6. Add the almonds to pan and bake for an additional 5 minutes or until almonds are browned.
7. Melt the butter in a large saucepan over medium heat setting.
8. Add onion and garlic and cook 4 minutes and stir occasionally.
9. Add apple and cook 3 minutes.
10. Add the curry powder and cook for 2 minutes and stir frequently.
11. Add the Cauliflower, almonds, 4 cups of water, salt, pepper, and bay leaf and allow it to boil.
12. Cover and cook 30 minutes or until Cauliflower and apple are very soft.
13. Discard bay leaf.
14. Place half of soup in a blender and blend until it turns smooth.
15. Pour it into a large bowl and repeat procedure with the remaining soup.
16. Return the soup to the pan and add the half-and-half.

17. Serve and top the soup with yogurt and chives then sprinkle with cracked black pepper.

Classic Chicken Noodle Soup

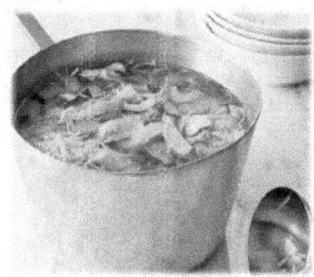

Classic Chicken Noodle Soup is what the doctor ordered any time of year! Bone-in chicken fortifies commercial stock and adds meaty depth to this Classic Chicken Noodle Soup.

PREP TIME: 28 mins

TOTAL TIME: 55 mins

YIELD: Serves 6 (serving size: about 1 cup)

Classic Chicken Noodle Soup

Ingredients
2 tablespoons of Canola oil
1 bone-in skinned chicken breast half
1 pound of skinned bone-in chicken thigh
¾ teaspoon of divided kosher salt
½ teaspoon of black pepper, divided
2 cups of chopped onion
1 cup of chopped carrot
½ cup (¼ -inch-thick) of sliced celery
1 tablespoon of minced fresh garlic
3 fresh parsley sprigs
3 fresh thyme sprigs
1 fresh rosemary sprig
2 bay leaves
1 cup of dry white wine

4 cups of unsalted chicken stock
1 cup of uncooked medium egg noodles
2 tablespoons of chopped fresh parsley

Preparation

1. Heat the oil in a Dutch oven over medium-high heat setting.
2. Sprinkle chicken with ½ teaspoon of salt and ¼ teaspoon of pepper.
3. Add the chicken with flesh side down.
4. Cook for 10 minutes and turn thigh after 5 minutes.
5. Let it Cool down and shred then discard the bones.
6. Add the onion, carrot, and celery to pan and cook for 10 minutes.
7. Add the garlic and cook for 1 minute.
8. Place the herb sprigs and bay leaves on cheesecloth.
9. Gather the edges and tie securely.
10. Add the sachet to pan, add wine, then boil it.
11. Cook for 4 minutes and add the chicken and the stock.
12. Cover it and reduce the heat and Cook for 7 minutes.
13. Add the noodles and cook 6 minutes or until al dente.
14. Discard the sachet and add the chopped parsley, the remaining ¼ teaspoon of salt, and remaining ¼ teaspoon of pepper.

Turkey Meatball Soup With Greens

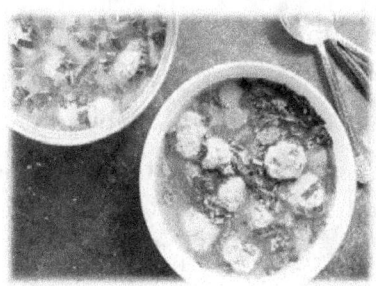

We like the softness of lacinato kale, but you can substitute other varieties in this soup.

PREP TIME: 40 mins

TOTAL TIME: 1 hour

YIELD: Serves 6

Turkey Meatball Soup with Greens

Ingredients
1-pound of grinded turkey breast
½ cup of cooked quinoa
2 ounces of grated and divided Parmigiano-Reggiano cheese, (about ½ cup)
2 tablespoons of chopped fresh flat-leaf parsley
2 tablespoons of chopped fresh basil
¾ teaspoon of divided kosher salt,
½ teaspoon of freshly divided grinded black pepper
6 minced and divided garlic cloves
1 lightly beaten large egg
4 teaspoons of divided extra-virgin olive oil
½ cup of chopped shallots
½ cup of chopped celery
8 cups of trimmed chopped lacinato kale (about 1 pound)

¼ teaspoon of crushed red pepper
5 cups of unsalted chicken stock
Lemon wedges (optional)

Preparation

1. Add the turkey, quinoa, ¼ cup cheese, parsley, basil, ¼ teaspoon of salt, ¼ teaspoon of black pepper, 2 garlic cloves, and egg in a large bowl then mix gently.
2. Shape the turkey mixture (about 2 tablespoons of each) into 24 meatballs with the damps in your hand.
3. Heat a large Dutch oven over medium-HIGH heat setting.
4. Add 1 teaspoon of oil to a pan and swirl to coat.
5. Add 12 meatballs and cook for 8 minutes, while turning them to brown on all sides.
6. Remove from the meatball from the pan and Repeat procedure with 1 teaspoon of oil and remaining 12 meatballs.
7. Add the remaining 2 teaspoons of oil to the pan and swirl to coat.
8. Add the shallots and celery to the oil in the pan and cook for 5 minutes.
9. Add the remaining 4 garlic cloves and cook for 1 minute.
10. Add kale, remaining ½ teaspoon of salt, remaining ¼ teaspoon of black pepper, and red pepper and cook 2 minutes and stir occasionally.
11. Add the stock and then allow it to boil.
12. Return the meatballs into pan and Reduce the heat then cook for 10 minutes or until the kale is soft and meatballs are done.
13. Serve 1 1/3 cups of soup into each of 6 bowls and divide the remaining cheese evenly among bowls.
14. Serve with lemon, if desired.

Mini Meatball Minestrone

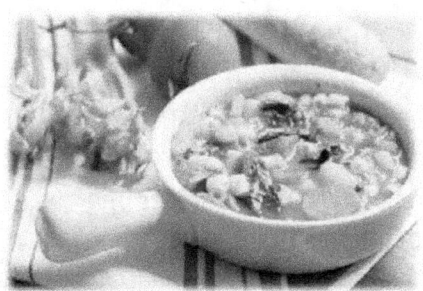

Don't take this soup lightly. Packed with mini meatballs, lettuce, tomatoes and chickpeas this hearty bowl of soup will not disappoint your taste buds.

PREP TIME: 25 mins

TOTAL TIME: 1 hour 25 mins

YIELD: Serves 8 (serving size: 1 cup of soup and about 4 meatballs)

Mini Meatball Minestrone

Ingredients
Soup:

1 tablespoon of olive oil
2 cups of diced onion
¾ cup (½ -inch) of sliced carrot
¾ cup (½ -inch) of sliced celery
¾ cup (½ -inch) of cubed parsnip
2 minced garlic cloves
3 cups of chopped Swiss chard
1 cup dry red wine
½ teaspoon of freshly grinded black pepper
¼ teaspoon of kosher salt
1 (32-ounce) container low heater-sodium beef broth

1 (14.5-ounce) CAN of no-salt-added diced tomatoes with basil, garlic, and oregano

Mini meatballs:

1-pound of grinded turkey
3 tablespoons of dry breadcrumbs
1 tablespoon of chopped fresh basil
1 tablespoon of olive oil
½ teaspoon of freshly grinded black pepper
¼ teaspoon of kosher salt
1 large egg, lightly beaten

Remaining ingredients:

1 (15-ounce) can of rinsed and drained chickpeas (garbanzo beans),
¼ cup chopped fresh basil
1 ounce grated fresh Parmesan cheese (optional)

Preparation

To prepare soup

1. Heat a large Dutch oven over medium-high heat setting.
2. Add the oil and swirl to coat.
3. Add the onion and the next 4 ingredients (through garlic) and cook for 6 minutes or the until vegetables are soft.
4. Add the chard and f cook for 1 minute or until it is wilted.
5. Add wine and the next 4 ingredients (through tomatoes).
6. Allow it to boil then reduce heat and cook for 10 minutes.

To prepare meatballs

1. Add the turkey and the next 6 ingredients (through egg) in a bowl.
2. Shape meat mixture with tablespoonful to make 30 meatballs.
3. Add the meatballs and the chickpeas to the soup.

4. Then boil over medium-high heat setting.
5. Cover it and cook for 12 minutes or until the meatballs are done.
6. Reduce the Heat and add ¼ cup of basil.
7. Serve the soup into bowls, and sprinkle evenly with Parmesan cheese, if desired.

Coconut Laksa With Shrimp

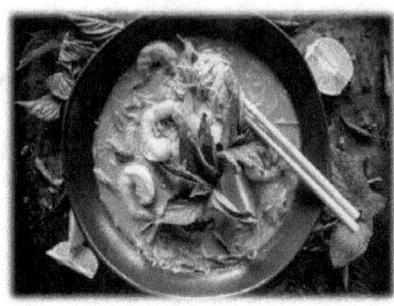

This hearty Southeast Asian noodle soup is sweet, spicy and vibrant, with a tropical creaminess from coconut milk.

PREP TIME: 1 hour

TOTAL TIME: 1 hour 30 mins

YIELD: 8 servings

Coconut Laksa with Shrimp

Ingredients

1 ½ pounds of shelled and deveined, shells reserved medium shrimp
1 quartered onion
1 sliced carrot
3 large quartered shallots
4 seeded and coarsely chopped jalapeños
1/3 cup of thinly sliced fresh ginger
¼ cup of macadamia nuts
1 teaspoon of grinded coriander
½ teaspoon of grinded turmeric
¼ cup of Asian fish sauce
¼ cup of Canola oil
2 plump of lemongrass stalks, bottom 8 inches only with the outer layer removed and stalk cut into 2-inch lengths

1 can of unsweetened coconut milk
2 tablespoons of light brown sugar
1 pound of Thai flat rice noodles (pad Thai), soaked in warm water for 10 minutes
Salt
Lime wedges, for serving

Preparation

1. Add the shrimp shells with the onion, carrot and 8 cups of water in a large saucepan and boil.
2. Cook over Moderate heat setting until the stock is bright orange in color and reduced to 5 cups, for about 30 minutes.
3. Strain and reserve the stock.
4. Add the shallots, jalapeños, ginger, macadamia nuts, coriander and turmeric with 2 tablespoons of the fish sauce and 2 tablespoons of the Canola oil, in a food processor, then blend until it is smooth.
5. Heat the remaining 2 tablespoons of oil in a soup pot.
6. Add the seasoning paste and cook over Moderate heat setting and stir, until the fragrant, is about 2 minutes.
7. Add the lemongrass and cook for about 10 minutes and stir occasionally, until the mixture darkens slightly and the oil separates.
8. Add the reserved shrimp stock, coconut milk, brown sugar and the remaining 2 tablespoons of fish sauce and Cook over Moderate heat setting until the soup is reduced to 6 cups, for about 15 minutes.
9. Meanwhile, cook the rice noodles until it is pliable in a large pot of boiling water, for about 1 minute.
10. Drain, while shaking out the excess water then transfer it to 8 soup bowls.

11. Add the shrimp to the soup and cook until it turns pink and curled, for about 5 minutes.
12. Season the soup with the salt and Serve it over the noodles.
13. Garnish with lime wedges and serve.

Chicken-And-Prosciutto Tortelloni Soup

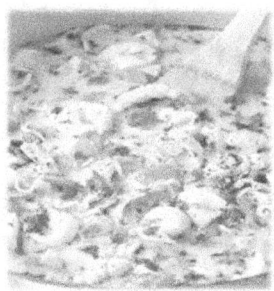

Any flavor tortelloni will work well in this dish.

PREP TIME: 20 mins

TOTAL TIME: 20 mins

YIELD: Makes 2 quarts

Chicken-and-Prosciutto Tortelloni Soup

Ingredients

1 (8-oz.) package of fresh chopped onions, peppers, and celery
1 tablespoon of olive oil
1/2 teaspoon of Italian seasoning
1 (14.5-oz.) can of diced tomatoes with roasted garlic
5 cups of reduced-sodium chicken broth
1/4 teaspoon of table salt
1/2 teaspoon of grinded black pepper
1 (9-oz.) package of refrigerated chicken-and-prosciutto tortelloni
1 (6-oz.) package of fresh baby spinach

Preparation

1. Cook the onions, peppers, and celery in hot oil in a Dutch oven over medium-high heat setting for 3 minutes.
2. Add the Italian seasoning, and cook for 1 minute.

3. Add the tomatoes and the next 3 ingredients then increase the heat to high heat setting, allow it to boil.
4. Add the tortelloni, and allow it to boil as well.
5. Reduce heat to low heat setting, and cook for 8 minutes or until the tortellini is soft.
6. Reduce the Heat, and add the spinach.

Southern Italian Chicken Soup

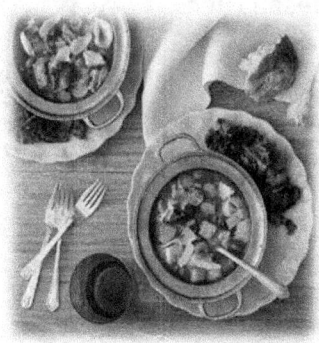

This simple pasta dish gets some savory Southern flare with the addition of okra and black-eyed peas. In just under an hour, this succulent soup comes together for a flavorful autumn or winter favorite.

PREP TIME: 45 mins

TOTAL TIME: 50 mins

YIELD: 8 servings

Southern Italian Chicken Soup

Ingredients

1 diced large onion
1 thinly sliced celery rib,
2 chopped carrots
1 minced garlic clove
3 tablespoons of divided olive oil
6 cups of chicken broth
1 (15.5-oz.) can of diced tomatoes
1 teaspoon dried Italian seasoning
1/4 teaspoon of dried crushed red pepper
4 (6- to 8-oz.) of skinned and boned chicken breasts
1/2 teaspoon of salt
1/2 teaspoon of black pepper

2 cups of sliced fresh okra
1 (15.5-oz.) can have drained and rinsed black-eyed peas
1 (9-oz.) package of refrigerated cheese-filled tortellini
Freshly grated Parmesan cheese

Preparation

1. Cook the first 4 ingredients in 2 Tbsp. of hot oil, in a large Dutch oven over medium-high heat setting for 3 to 5 minutes or until it is soft.
2. Add the broth and the next 3 ingredients then boil and stir occasionally.
3. Reduce the heat to medium, and cook and stir occasionally for 10 minutes.
4. Meanwhile, sprinkle the chicken with salt and black pepper and cook the remaining 1 Tbsp. of hot oil in a large nonstick skillet, Over Medium-high heat setting for 5 minutes on each side or until it is lightly browned.
5. Let it cool down slightly for about 5 minutes then cut it into 1-inch pieces.
6. Add the okra, black-eyed peas, and chicken to Dutch oven.
7. Cook and stir occasionally for 10 minutes or until the okra is soft.
8. Add the tortellini, and cook and stir for 3 minutes or until tortellini is done.
9. Serve with Parmesan.

Amish Style Chicken And Corn Soup

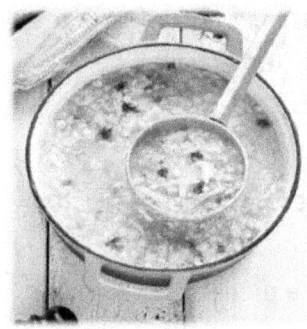

This delicious chicken and corn soup will fill you up and keep you warm and toasty on a cold fall day. This recipe is a traditional Amish staple. The best thing about Amish cooking is that it uses very simple, natural ingredients, and this chicken soup recipe is no exception. The ingredients provide a sweet and savory flavor combination that you're sure to love. It's easy to make this great soup for the whole family!

PREP TIME: 45 mins

TOTAL TIME: 50 mins

YIELD: 8 servings

Amish Style Chicken and Corn Soup

Ingredients

½ stewing hen
2 quarts of chicken stock or broth
¼ cup of coarsely chopped onion
½ cup of coarsely chopped carrots
½ cup of coarsely chopped celery
1 teaspoon of saffron threads (optional)
¾ cup corn kernels
½ cup of finely chopped celery
1 tablespoon of chopped fresh parsley,

1 cup of cooked egg noodles

Preparation

1. Combine the stewing hen with the chicken stock, coarsely chopped onions, carrots, celery, and saffron threads and cook them altogether.
2. Cook for about 1 hour, while skimming the surface as necessary.
3. Remove and reserve the stewing hen until if I done, then separate the meat from the bones.
4. Cut into neat, little pieces.
5. Then Strain the saffron broth through a fine sieve.
6. Add the corn, celery, parsley, and the cooked noodles to the broth.
7. Cook the soup again and serve immediately.

Chicken And Dumplings Soup

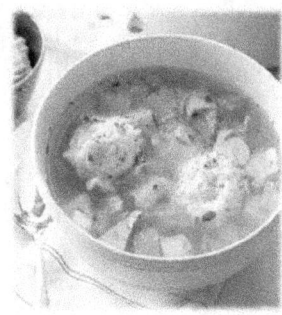

This is the perfect filling soup for a cold weather day. This chicken recipe is hearty and soothing. This is a classic comforting chicken soup flavor that is at the base of this dish. Plus, the homemade dumplings are so delicious that you won't be able to resist this easy soup recipe. It is so good that you will be feeling better in no time!

Chicken and Dumplings Soup

Ingredients

Soup:
1 whole chicken
1 or two chopped celery ribs or leaves
1 chopped carrot
1 chopped onion
Water to cover
2 tablespoons of butter

Dumplings:
2 cups of flour
2 teaspoons of baking powder
½ teaspoon of salt
1 cup of whole milk

4 tablespoons of vegetable oil
Preparation

Soup:

1. Cook the chicken with celery, carrot, and onion in water to cover, until the meat is separated from the bone.
2. Take the chicken out of the broth and set aside.
3. Remove the celery, carrot, and onion, then strain the broth and pour the broth into a Dutch oven or large pot.
4. Separate the chicken from the bone and return it into the soup.
5. Add butter and Bring boil the soup.
6. While soup is heating up, mix the dumplings

Dumplings:

7. Mix the ingredients, blend it well, and turn it out onto a floured surface.
8. Knead 4 or 5 times and Roll out the dough to ⅛ inch thick and cut into 1 x 1 ½ inch strips.
9. Drop the strip one at a time into soup.
10. Reduce the heat to medium-low and cover it for 15 minutes.
11. Break dumplings to smaller particles if you like and sprinkle with pepper.
12. return the cover back on, but do not turn the heat back on.
13. Wait for 30 minutes then serve and enjoy.

Debra's Cauliflower Soup

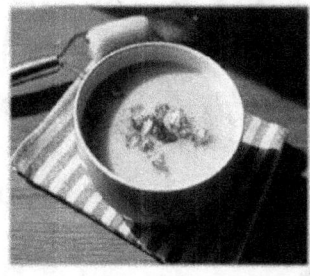

For a delicious, belly-warming soup, you need got to try this Debra's cauliflower soup! It is cheesy, zippy, and simply divine. You can easily change the recipe to make this a vegetarian recipe, but the ham adds a hearty, meaty touch. Plus, the mildness of the Muenster cheese makes the cauliflower in the soup come to life in your mouth. Now, don't hesitate! Make a batch of this creamy soup today and serve it up with your favorite rolls.

Debra's Cauliflower Soup

Ingredients
1 whole head of cauliflower
2 cups of chicken stock
1 cup of milk
3 tablespoons of cornstarch
1 cup of diced ham
2 cloves of garlic
2 tablespoons of olive oil
½ tablespoon of Worcestershire sauce to taste
salt and pepper, to taste
8 deli slices of Muenster cheese
Preparation

1. Cook the cauliflower in chicken stock for 30 minutes (no need to chop, cauliflower, it will collapse when you stir in other ingredients).
2. Mince the 2 garlic cloves and add 2 tablespoons of olive oil.
3. Add the diced ham and cook until it is heated through, while stirring with garlic cloves.
4. Add the cornstarch to milk and add the ham mixture.
5. Heat until it becomes bubbling, while stirring gently, and add it to the cauliflower and chicken stock.
6. Stir when it boils for about 1 minute, then add the seasonings and cheese.
7. Heat on warm heat settings for about 5 more minutes until the cheese has melted, then stir as necessary.
8. Serve with warm rolls or any bread of choice.

www.ingramcontent.com/pod-product-compliance
Lightning Source LLC
Chambersburg PA
CBHW071441070526
44578CB00001B/177